Coronary Heart
Disease in
Clinical Practice

Coronary Heart Disease in Clinical Practice

Satish Mittal

With 14 Figures, 2 in Full Color

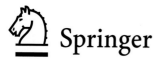 Springer

Satish Mittal, MBBS
General Medical Practitioner (formerly, General Practice Principal, East Molesey, East Surrey Health Authority, Surrey, UK; and Clinical Governance Lead cum Chairman Clinical Governance Committee, East Elmbridge Primary Care Group, Esher, Surrey, UK)

Cover illustration: Courtesy of Vahini V. Naidoo, MD, Consultant in Nuclear Cardiology, Hon. Senior Lecturer, Imperial College, Royal Brompton Hospital, London.

British Library Cataloguing in Publication Data
A catalogue record for this book is available from the British Library

Library of Congress Control Number: 2005923549

ISBN-10: 1-85233-936-5   e-ISBN 1-84628-135-0
ISBN-13: 978-1-85233-936-4

Springer Science+Business Media
springeronline.com

Typeset by SNP Best-set Typesetter Ltd., Hong Kong
Printed in the United States of America
28-543210 Printed on acid-free paper

In memory of my father,
Harish Chandra,
and my mother,
Ramanandi

Foreword

Dr. Satish Mittal has produced a single authored book entitled, *Coronary Heart Disease in Clinical Practice*. In it, he has reviewed several clinical topics that are important in evaluation and treatment of patients with coronary heart disease. Topics reviewed include risk factors, diabetes, hypertension, coronary interventions, heart failure, and arrhythmias. The acute coronary syndromes are discussed and a "Healthy Life Style" is reviewed. In each chapter, key clinical studies are summarized and recommendations for treatment are developed. Questions pertaining to specific clinical problems and their answers are also provided in the text of each discussion. The single focus of the book, the reviews of clinical studies, and the useful clinical approach that is provided for the care of each of these problems should be helpful to all who care for patients with this very important problem.

James T. Willerson, MD
President, The University of Texas Health Science Center at Houston
President-Elect and Medical Director, Texas Heart Institute

About This Book

Coronary heart disease is increasingly common and is the single largest preventable and treatable cause of mortality worldwide. *Coronary Heart Disease in Clinical Practice* is a concise and thorough reference book directed at medical practitioners, clinicians, practice nurses, medical students, and those in associated fields. The information is presented in an accessible question-and-answer format. It highlights important aspects of numerous current guidelines, making this a valuable, timesaving reference tool that incorporates the latest research in the field.

The broad coverage of this book includes chapters on coronary heart disease, its risk factors (lipids, hypertension, diabetes, and lifestyle), and coronary events (angina, acute myocardial infarction, heart failure, and arrhythmias). The text contains carefully selected, complex discussions on medical hot topics. Each topic is explained at length with the aid of illustrations and tables. In a book of this size I have endeavoured to include most of the important relevant issues pertaining to coronary heart disease in clinical practice. In doing so I have adhered to the widely accepted guidelines on various important issues in clinical medicine. I have mentioned the pharmaceutical preparations by generic names only and have not included combination preparations for which the reader should refer to the particular pharmaceutical preparations.

I am thankful to my son Ajay for contributing the tables and illustrations.

Contents

Chapter 1
Healthy Living

Healthy living constitutes an integral part of preventing coronary heart disease (CHD). It lowers the risk of CHD both in free-living, high-risk patients and in cardiac patients. The combined effect of a healthy diet and lifestyle factors is larger than their individual effects. Trials based on both primary prevention in high-risk patients and secondary prevention in cardiac patients show that there is substantial reduction in the risk of CHD by suitable diet and lifestyle changes. Cholesterol lowering is not the only route through which diet can influence the occurrence of CHD in cardiac patients. Dietary changes that influence other metabolic pathways can also be beneficial.

NUTRITION

Adequate diet is very important from birth and throughout life. Dietary management also plays a crucial role in the prevention of CHD. Up to 30% of all deaths from CHD have been attributed to unhealthy diet.[1] An atherogenic diet should be avoided. Important constituents of adequate diet include antioxidants, folic acid, other B vitamins, omega-3 fatty acids, and other nutrients. One gram of fat, 1 g of carbohydrates, and protein supply 9 kcal (38 kJ), 3.75 kcal (16 kJ), and 4 kcal (17 kJ), respectively. The Lifestyle Heart Trial[2] demonstrated coronary plaque regression (−1.75%) and a reduction in the number of anginal episodes at 1 year in a small group of 28 people with CHD who were able to make a comprehensive range of lifestyle changes.

Q: What are the main dietary constituents that are relevant in the context of CHD?
These are as follows:

Fats

Fats are broken down during digestion into fatty acids and glycerol, which are absorbed into the blood, to be used either immediately to provide energy or to be stored as energy reserve. Fatty acids may be unsaturated or saturated. The unsaturated may be monosaturated (omega-9) or polyunsaturated (i.e., omega-6 [linoleic acid] or omega-3 [alpha-linolenic acid]). Fatty acids can also be described according to their chain (e.g., C16, C18), and then adding the number of double bonds after a colon (e.g., 16:0, C18: 1).

Saturated Fatty Acids (SFAs)
High intake of SFAs is associated with increased population rates of CHD. Some saturated fatty acids are more harmful than others. Myristic acid (C14:0) is most harmful. Palmitic acid (C16) is less harmful than myristic acid. Those containing a longer chain (stearic acid, C18:0) and those containing a shorter one (C12 or less) seem to be less harmful. Saturates from C12 to C16 chain lengths have been directly linked to the elevation in low-density lipoprotein (LDL) cholesterol, although the evidence for C12:0 (lauric acid) is less clear. Rich sources of saturated fats are fatty meat, poultry skin, full-fat dairy foods, butter, ghee, palm oil, palm kernel oil, and coconut oil. Foods high in saturated fat, *trans*-fat, and cholesterol are lard and meat.

Trans-Fatty Acids
Trans-fatty acids are those in which double bonds are in the *trans* configuration. They are usually produced by hydrogenation of vegetable oils, but some quantities are also found naturally in animal fats. *Trans*-fatty acids raise the LDL-C level, and their high intake is associated with increased CHD risk. *Trans*-fatty acids are not classified as saturated fatty acids, and are not included in the quantitative recommendation of SFA intake of less than 7%. Their intake should be kept very low. Rich sources of these fatty acids are products made from partially hydrogenated oils, such as crackers, cookies, doughnuts, breads, French fries, and chicken fried in hydrogenated shortening. Soft margarines and vegetable oil spreads have low amounts.

Monounsaturated Fatty Acids (MUFAs)
Monounsaturated fatty acids are now promoted as the main source of dietary fat because of their lower susceptibility to lipid peroxidation and consequently lower atherogenic potential. It has been clearly shown that oleic acid (18:1 *cis*) has a powerful affect in lowering LDL and triglycerides, and it probably also increases the level of high-density lipoprotein (HDL). The low incidence of ischemic heart disease in the Mediterranean region is thought to be due

to dietary intake of oleic acid. Olive oil spread from olive oil and rapeseed/groundnut/canola oils are the richest source of *cis*-monosaturated fatty acid. Rapeseed oil, now available cheaply throughout Europe, is rich in oleic acid. Other sources are avocado and most nuts. Most MUFAs should be derived from vegetable sources including plant oils and nuts. The benefit of replacing SFA with MUFA has not been properly tested in trials.

Polyunsaturated Fatty Acids (PUFAs)
Linoleic acid (C18: 2,n-6) and alpha-linolenic acid (C18: 33,n-3) are essential fatty acids. They cannot be synthesized in the body and therefore should be included in the diet. Other long chain fatty acids of importance are arachidonic (C20: 4,n-6), eicosapentenoic (C20: 5,n-3), and docosahexaenoic acid (C22: 6,n-3). These can be synthesized in the body from linoleic and alpha-linolenic. When substituted for saturated acids, they cause some reduction of total cholesterol and triglycerides. PUFAs are one form of unsaturated fatty acids that can replace saturated fat. Most PUFAs should be derived from liquid oils and semiliquid margarines. Recommended intake should be up to 12% of total calories.

Omega-6 Fatty Acids (Linoleic Acid 18:2: n–6)
These fatty acids reduce the level of cholesterol, LDL, and frequently triglycerides in the blood. If fewer amounts are taken in the diet, the level of LDL tends to rise, and there is an increased risk of thrombosis. People of higher social class tend to consume less. Its level is also reduced among smokers. Rich sources of omega-6 are corn oil, sunflower, safflower, and soya bean oil, spreads derived from these oils, and seeds (Table 1.1).

Trials have suggested that a high polyunsaturated/saturated ratio due to omega-6 fatty acids supplementation in diet was associated with a reduced risk of ischemic heart disease. These fatty acids also have an antithrombotic effect. Intake should be less than 10% of energy. Consumption of omega-6 has increased considerably recently and now comprises 6% of food energy. No further increase is currently recommended until the safety of a higher intake of over 10% has been evaluated. Ideally, people should replace saturates with some monosaturates and some polyunsaturates.

Omega-3 Fatty Acids (Alpha-Linolenic 18:3: n–3)
Alpha-linolenic acid primarily occurs in vegetable sources such as soya bean, canola oil, English walnuts, and eicosapentaenoic acid (EPA; C20:5) and docosahexaenoic acid (DHA; C22:6) in marine

TABLE 1.1. The percentage of fatty acids in different food components

	Saturated	Oleic	Linoleic
Polyunsaturated margarine	18	20	50
Butter	69	28	3
Sunflower oil	12	25	63
Corn oil	12	30	54
Beef fat	51	39	2
Lard (pork)	39	45	10
Rapeseed oil	7	62	31
Olive oil	14	76	9
Soya bean oil	15	64	20
Palm oil	45	45	9
Lamb	50	38	4
Pork	42	50	7

Note: Oleic acid is monosaturated, and linoleic acid is polyunsaturated.

fish and fish oils. Omega-3 intake derived from both plant and marine sources reduce sudden death and overall death in people with preexisting cardiovascular disease (CVD). Omega-3 is antithrombogenic and hypotriglyceridemic; it reduces the growth of atherogenic plaque; it reduces adhesion molecule expression and platelet-derived growth factor; it is antiinflammatory; it promotes nitric oxide–induced endothelial function; and it is mildly hypotensive.[3] It also prevents arrhythmia and probably inhibits cyclooxygenase (COX), though the effect is not as potent as that of aspirin. The epidemiological evidence is not entirely consistent, but, like linoleic acid, there is an inverse relation between eicosapentaenoic acid and angina and heart attack. Eating fish twice a week reduces the risk of cardiac mortality. It also seems to reduce the progression of atheroma formation in coronary arteries and prevents restenosis after revascularization procedures.

Unlike the omega-6 type, omega-3 fatty acids do not reduce the level of total or low-density lipoproteins. The richest source is oily fish and marine oils. Other sources are wheat, rapeseed, green vegetables (e.g., spinach), and certain oils (e.g., soya bean and rapeseed oils). The alpha-linolenic acid content of various vegetable oils (per teaspoonful) is as follows: olive oil, 0.1 g; English walnut, 0.7 g; soya bean, 0.9 g; canola oil, 1.3 g; walnut oil, 1.4 g; flax seeds, 2.2 g; flax seed oil (linseed) oil, 8.5 g.[4] The current average intake of omega-3 is 0.1 g/day. It is recommended that this intake be doubled to 0.2 g/day.

It is shown that people at risk of CHD benefit from consumption of plant- and marine-derived omega-3 fatty acids. Evidence from prospective secondary studies suggests that EPA and DHA supplementation ranging from 0.5 to 1.8 g/d (either as fatty fish or supplement) significantly reduces subsequent cardiac and all-cause mortality. For alpha-linolenic acid, a total intake of 1.5 to 3 g/d seems to be beneficial. Both plant-based (alpha-linolenic acid) and fish-based (EPA and DHA) supplements have shown benefits in secondary coronary artery disease (CAD) prevention. In the GISSI-Prevenzione trial of 11,324 postinfarction patients in Italy, the effects of adding vitamin E (300 mg) and/or n-3 polyunsaturated fatty acids (capsule containing 850 mg) to the diet were studied. After 3.5 years, the patients randomized to receive fish oil capsules had a reduction in vascular risk of 15% in the composite primary end point of total mortality, nonfatal myocardial infarction (MI), and stroke. The relative risk of cardiovascular death was reduced by 30% and of sudden death by 45%. These benefits were apparent after just 4 months.[5] The Diet and Reinfarction Trial (DART) found that those subjects randomized to receive the advice to eat more fish had a greater survival rate.[6] This was a relatively large secondary prevention trial in which subjects were advised to eat oily fish twice a week. The subjects had a 32% reduction in CHD mortality and 29% reduction in 2-year all-cause mortality compared with a control group that was not advised. Examples of oily (fatty) fish are herring, kipper, pilchards, salmon (tinned or fresh), sardines, trout, fresh tuna (not tinned), whitebait, mackerel, sprats or brisling, and white bait (Table 1.2).

Various studies suggest that consumption of fish and of highly UFA food in general (and omega-3 fatty acids in particular) reduced the risk of CHD. In a study monitoring 22,071 men with no prior CHD for up to 17 years, higher baseline blood levels of n-3 fatty acids (FAs) were strongly associated with a reduced risk of sudden death even after controlling for confounding factors.[7] In secondary prevention trials, increased consumption of fatty fish or dietary supplement n-3 FA led to a reduction in coronary events.[8] American Heart Association (AHA) recommendation for the intake of omega-3 fatty acids are as follows:

- Patients without proven CHD should eat fish (preferably oily) at least twice a week, and should include oils and foods rich in alpha-linolenic acid in their diets.
- Patients with CHD should take 1 g of EPA and DHA daily, preferably from fish oil. Supplementation could be considered on the advice of their physicians.
- Patients with hypertriglyceridemia should take 2 to 4 g of EPA daily, provided as capsules under medical supervision.

TABLE 1.2. EPA and DHA content (g)/100 g of edible fish

Fish	EPA + DHA content
Tuna (fresh)	0.25–1.51
Salmon	1.28–2.15
Mackerel	0.4–1.85
Halibut	0.47–1.18
Cod	0.28
Haddock	0.24
Oyster	0.44
Scallop	0.2
Atlantic herring	2.01
Trout	1.15
Sardines	1.15–2
Tuna (canned)	0.31
Catfish	0.18
Flounder	0.45
Shrimp	0.32

EPA, eicosapentaenoic acid; DHA, docosahexaenoic acid. Data from USDA Nutrient Data Laboratory www.nalusda.gov/fnic/foodcomp.

A U.S. panel of nutritional scientists has recommended an intake of EPA and DHA 0.65 g/d, whereas the British Nutrition Foundation's recommendation is 1.2 g/d.

A vegetarian diet, especially that of vegans, is relatively low in alpha-linolenic acid and provides little if any EPA and DHA. Clinical studies suggest that tissue levels of long-chain n-3 fatty acids are depressed in vegetarians, and particularly in vegans. Therefore, total n-3 requirements may be higher for vegetarians than for nonvegetarians, as vegetarians must rely on conversion of alpha-linolenic acid to EPA and DHA. Information is available at www.nutrition.org.uk (accessed 1.21.05).

Carbohydrates

The main function of carbohydrates is to provide energy, but they are also important for various metabolic processes. Carbohydrates may be classified as sugars and polysaccharides. Polysaccharides are of two types: starch polysaccharides (complex carbohydrates) and nonstarch polysaccharides (NSP). Sugar intake should be reduced while the complex carbohydrate intake should increase. The organization Diabetes UK advocates that there is no scientific basis for making a distinction between starches and sugars, as the body handles them both in the same way. Both provide 4 kcal and are potentially caloriogenic, the glycemic effects of both are similar, and both are generally eaten in composite foods that supply other nutrients.

Complex Carbohydrates

Recommended carbohydrate intake is up to 60% of total calories, but in a patient with metabolic syndrome it should be restricted to 50%. These carbohydrates are contained in whole wheat bread, whole grain rice, whole wheat pastry, potatoes, leafy vegetables, root vegetables, millet, sun-dried fruit, fresh fruit, oats, barley, rye, nuts, seeds, lentils, beans, and chick peas. Most carbohydrates should be derived from grain products, especially whole grain, vegetables, and fruits, and fat-free and low-fat dairy products.

Fiber (Nonstarch Polysaccharides)

Fiber is of three types:

- Cellulose, which is contained in the cell wall and cannot be broken down, is not absorbed. It is insoluble in water. Rich sources are leafy vegetables, peas, beans, and rhubarb.
- Lignin, like cellulose, is contained in the cell wall, and is also not broken down in the gut, but it constitutes a small part of food content. It is also insoluble.
- Noncellulose is of either the soluble type (oat, barley, seeds [especially phylum], rye, fruit, vegetables, wheat) or the insoluble type (mushrooms, leafy vegetables, peas, beans, rhubarb). Viscous (soluble) fiber helps to reduce LDL-C, whereas the insoluble type does not significantly affect it. Five to 10 g/d of viscous fiber reduces LDL-C by approximately 5%. One gram of soluble fiber is provided by a half cup of cooked barley, oatmeal, or oat bran, whereas a half cup of phylum seeds (ground) provides 5 g. A half cup of cooked beans provides 2 to 3 g, a half cup of lentils, peas, broccoli, or carrots provide 1 g, and a half cup of brussels sprouts provides 3 g. One medium-size fruit (apple, banana, nectarine, plum) provides 1 g of soluble fiber, and one citrus fruit or pear provides 2 g.[9]

Proteins

Proteins are composed of amino acids. Plant protein alone can provide enough of the essential and nonessential amino acids. Soya protein has been shown to be equal to protein of animal sources. Protein has little effect on LDL-C but substituting soya protein for animal protein has been reported to lower LDL-C. Proteins are mainly found in meat, fish, cheese, milk, other dairy products, poultry, eggs, beans, lentils, and nuts. In 1999, the U.S. Food and Drug Administration (FDA) approved claims that 25 g/d of soya protein reduces heart disease. Soya intake causes reduction of total cholesterol by 9.3%, LDL-C by 12.9% and triglycerides by 10.5%, and increases HDL-C by 2.4%.

Consumption of nuts is consistently associated with an inverse CHD risk in prospective studies. Nuts are high in unsaturated fat. Most nuts are associated with changes in lipid/lipoprotein that reduce CHD risk. The association may be related to various constituents in the nuts such as MUFAs, PUFAs, vitamin E, arginine precursors, flavoniods, and other polyphenols. Diet supplementation with walnuts and almonds reduce total and LDL-C. In the Nurses Health Study (1998), 89,409 nurses were followed for 14 years. One nurse in 20 ate five or more helpings of nuts a week. In this group, the CHD risk was reduced by 35% compared with the one third of the nurses who did not eat nuts.

Q: What is the dietary recommendation for sodium and potassium?

Sodium
Increased intake of sodium contributes to hypertension. A typical diet contains far more sodium than recommended; between two thirds and four fifths come from manufactured foods, with the remainder being added during cooking or at the table. The average intake should be reduced by a third from 9 g/d to 6 g/d (100 mmol or 2.4 g Na). Foods that are rich in salt are potato chips, salted nuts, and canned, preserved, and processed foods. The amount of sodium that is labeled in food packages as "g/100 g" can be converted into salt measured in grams by multiplying the figure by 2.5.

Potassium
It is recommended that the average intake of potassium should be increased from 2 to 3 g/d to 2 to 4 g/d. Several prospective population studies have shown reduced stroke incidence and mortality with increased dietary potassium. In Finland, "Pansuola," a modified table salt, has been introduced; it is composed of 57% NaCl, 28% KCl, 12% $MgSO_4$, 2% L-lysine, and anticaking agent. Using Pansuola, sodium intake is reduced by 30% to 50% with improvement in the sodium/potassium ratio. The main sources of potassium are meat, cereal, milk, bananas, beetroot, melon, oranges, potatoes, cabbage, butter, beans, figs, nuts (not salted), grapefruit, grapes, and dates. Most vegetables and fruits are moderately rich in potassium.

Q: What are the current dietary recommendations based on present studies?

The Mediterranean diet is low in saturated fat and high in unsaturated fat, whereas the traditional Japanese diet is low in saturated fat but rich in complex carbohydrates. Both diets are good, though the Mediterranean is more lipid friendly and cardioprotective. Recent dietary trials in secondary prevention of CHD have produced impressive results, with a reduction of recurrence rates by a range of 30% to 70%, because, unlike previous trials, these diets were characterized by a low intake of total and saturated fats and/or an increased intake of marine or plant n-3 fatty acids, and they were not intended primarily to reduce blood cholesterol.

The Lyon Diet Heart Study is a randomized secondary prevention trial of 302 experimental and 303 control subjects, aimed at testing whether a Mediterranean-type diet (included alphalinolenic acid), as compared with a prudent Western-type diet, may reduce the rate of recurrence after the first MI. The experimental subjects consumed significantly fewer lipids, saturated fats, cholesterol, and linoleic acid, but more oleic acid and alpha-linoleic acid. They were allowed to use for salad dressing only rapeseed and olive oils. Alcohol was allowed in moderation. The diet was adapted to a Mediterranean-type diet: more bread, more root and green vegetables, more fish, less meat (beef, lamb, and pork were replaced with poultry), fruit every day, and margarine replaced butter and cream (Table 1.3).

TABLE 1.3. Essential components of different diets: recommended intake as percentage of total calories

Nutrients	Lyon diet	UK Diabetes*	Eating Plan for Healthy Americans	TLC diet total lifestyle change**
Total fat	30%	<35%	To meet calorie needs	25–35%
Saturates	8%	<10%	7–10%	<7%
Polyunsaturates	5%	10–20%	Up to 10%	Up to 10%
Monounsaturates	13%	<10%	Up to 15%	Up to 20%
Carbohydrates		45–60%	55% or more	50–60%
Protein	16.2%	<1 g/kg body wt	Approx. 15%	Approx. 15%
Cholesterol	203 mg/day	300 mg/day	<300 mg/day	<200 mg/day

* Also sucrose up to 10%, salt ≤6 g/d.
** Also, plant stanols/sterols 2 g/day, dietary fiber 20–30 g/d, viscous (soluble) fiber 10–25 g/d, salt ≤ 6.1 g/d (National Cholesterol Education Program, Adult Treatment Panel III).
TLC, Total Lifestyle Changes.[9]

After a mean follow-up of 27 months, there were 16 cardiac deaths in the control group and three in the experimental group; 17 nonfatal MI in controls and five in the experimental group. The risk ratio for these two main end points combined was 0.27 (95% confidence interval [CI] 0.12–0.59, $p = .001$) after adjustment for prognostic variables. The overall mortality was 20 in the controls and eight in the experimental group, and the adjusted risk ratio was 0.30 (95% CI 0.11–0.82, $p = .02$).[8] An alpha-linolenic acid–rich diet seems to be more effective than the subjects' previously used diet in secondary prevention. Although the study was planned for 5 years, its scientific and ethics committee terminated it at 27 months because the benefits were very favorable. The rate of cardiac death and nonfatal infarction in the experimental group after 46 months is similar to that at 27 months.[10]

The trial reinforced the cardioprotective effect of these foods, with particular emphasis on n-3 fatty acids and on folates for their role in hyperhomocysteinemia and in the arginine–nitric oxide–tetrahydrobiopterin pathway, two major mediators in the development of CHD. This trial emphasized that relatively simple dietary changes achieved greater reduction in the risk of all-cause and CHD mortality. Adherence to the traditional Mediterranean diet was associated with a reduction in the concentration of inflammatory and coagulation markers, and this may explain its beneficial action in the cardiovascular system.[11] Plant-based n-3 may particularly reduce CHD risk when seafood-based n-3 is low.[12]

In another study, patients who were suspected cases of MI were treated with fish oil capsules (EPA 1.08 g/d), mustard oil (alpha-linolenic acid 2.9 g/d), or placebo. After 1 year, total coronary events were significantly less in the group taking fish oil and mustard seed oil supplement.[13] The American Heart Association's Eating Plan for Healthy Americans is recommended for healthy people. The Step-II diet has been replaced by the Total Lifestyle Changes (TLC) diet, which is recommended for all people who have heart disease or are at increased risk.

Practical Advice on Dietary Intake

- Consume a variety of fruits, vegetables, and grain products, including whole grains, nuts, and legumes. Whole grains as well as nutrients fortified and enriched with starches, such as cereals, should be the major source of calories in the diet.
- Consume wholemeal bread (especially whole grain bread), root vegetables, and green vegetables. Eat five portions (≥400 g) of fruits and vegetables daily. One portion is equal to one medium apple, one medium banana, one orange, five apricots, two sat-

sumas, one medium tomato, three heaping tablespoons of beans, carrots, fruit salad, or peas, two spears of broccoli, one table-spoonful of raisins, and one cereal bowl of lettuce. Canned and frozen varieties are as good as fresh ones. For more information, go to www.doh.gov.uk/fiveaday/ (accessed 1.31.05).

- Foods rich in starches (polysaccharides, i.e., bread, pasta, cereals, potatos) are recommended over sugars.
- Replace saturated fatty acids and *trans*-fatty acids with unsaturated fats, especially with monosaturated and nonhydrogenated polysaturated fat.
- Replace butter with olive oil or monosaturated margarine (e.g., rapeseed or olive oil based). Avoid commercial bakery and deep fried foods (they contain high levels of *trans*-fats and sugars).
- Increased intake of omega-3 and omega-6 fatty acids. Increase omega-3 fatty acids from fish oil and plants. Higher dietary intake of n-3 fatty acids in the form of fatty fish or vegetable oils is an option for reducing the risk of CHD.
- Reduce salt intake (<6 g/d), especially for people with hypertension.
- Antioxidants should be taken from natural dietary sources.
- Alcohol intake is restricted to 2 units/d for women and 3 units/d for men.
- Increased dietary fiber, especially soluble fiber.
- Dietary cholesterol should be <300 mg/d in those without cardiovascular (CV) risk and <200 mg in those with CV risk.

Interpretation of Food Labels
- "Low fat" means 5 g or less of fat per 100 g of product.
- Reduced or "lower" fat means that the fat content has been reduced by 25% or more.
- "85% fat-free" means 15% of total weight is fat (i.e., 15 g of 100 g).

ALCOHOL
Alcohol intake is measured in terms of units. A U.K. unit is equal to 30 mL (1 fluid oz) of spirits (whisky, vodka, brandy), 300 mL (one half pint) of beer, or one glass (120 mL or 4 oz) of wine. Roughly, a bottle of spirits contains 30 units, and a bottle of wine contains seven units. Maximum recommended weekly intake of alcohol is 21 units (a maximum of three units per day) for men and 14 units (a maximum of two units per day) for women. This is better taken on a regular basis rather than as a one-day binge. Some alcohol-free days are also recommended. U.S. guidelines advise a maximum of two drinks (1 oz or 30 mL ethanol, e.g., 24 oz of beer, 10 oz of wine, or 3 oz of 80-proof whisky) per day for men and no more than

one drink per day for women. One gram of alcohol provides 7 kcal/g of energy. The legal limit for driving in the United Kingdom is 80 mg of alcohol in 100 mL of blood. On an average it takes 1 hour for the body to get rid of one unit of alcohol.

Q: Is alcohol cardioprotective?

Moderate daily intake of one to two drinks of alcohol is associated with a 30% to 40% lower risk of heart disease.[14,15] Moderate drinking is likely to have the most beneficial effects in people who are at highest risk of CHD, i.e., middle-aged and elderly people. There is no evidence that drinking when young confers protection later in life against coronary heart disease. Besides, much of the benefit of alcohol on coronary heart disease is seen in people at otherwise high risk. Excessive intake of alcohol is directly damaging to the myocardium, possibly through a mechanism involving the nonoxidative metabolism of ethanol to fatty acid ethyl ester.[16]

The pattern of drinking is also important. Drinking patterns have changed little among men over the last 10 years, but among women alcohol intake has increased. Consumption of excess alcohol on at least 3 to 4 days per week has been found to be inversely associated with the risk of heart attack in men.[17] Conversely, binge drinking is associated with increased mortality and fatal heart attack. There is some concern that moderate drinking may increase the risk of breast cancer in young women (<50 years). Heavy drinking predisposes to obesity, hypertension, arrhythmia, cardiomyopathy, and hemorrhagic stroke. It can cause a variety of other medical disorders (i.e., liver cirrhosis, upper gastrointestinal bleeding, depression, neuropathy, gout, infertility, and sexual problems).

Q: What is the mechanism of the cardioprotective effect of alcohol?

The mechanism of the cardioprotective effect of alcohol is complex, and is as follows:

- Increases the levels of HDL cholesterol, its subfractions HDL-2 and HDL-3, and apolipoproteins A-1 and A-41. Increases in HDL levels account for 50% of alcohol's cardioprotective effect.
- Reduces levels of inflammation.
- Improves insulin sensitivity, which may in turn be part of the reason for the favorable lipid profile.
- Affects the coagulation system by decreasing platelet aggregation and fibrinogen levels, thus reducing the risk of thrombosis. It also promotes clot lyses by increasing the release of plasminogen activator.[18]

exercise and is usually expressed in metabolic equivalents (METs). One MET, the energy expended by sitting quietly, is equivalent to 3.5 mL of oxygen uptake per kilogram of body weight per minute, or 1 kcal per kilogram body weight per hour. Relative intensity refers to the percentage of aerobic power utilized during exercise and is expressed as the percentage of maximum heart rate or percent of maximum oxygen consumption (Vo_2max). Moderate intensity exercises are those performed at a relative intensity of 40% to 60% of VO_2max (or absolute intensity of 4 to 6 METs). Vigorous intensity activities are performed at a relative intensity of >60% of Vo_2max (or absolute intensity of >6 METs)[25] (Table 1.5).

Following are the important advantages of exercise:

- Beneficial changes in hemodynamic, hormonal, metabolic, neurological, and respiratory function occur with increased exercise capacity.[26] Exercise training increases cardiovascular functional capacity and decreases myocardial oxygen demand at any level of physical activity in apparently healthy people as well as in most individuals with CVD.
- Exercise favorably alters lipids and carbohydrate metabolism, controls diabetes and obesity, and improves insulin sensitivity.
- Aerobic exercise reduces blood pressure 8 to 10 mm Hg (both systolic and diastolic).
- Exercise enhances the beneficial effects of a low saturated fat and low cholesterol diet on the blood.
- Endurance training has effects on adipose tissue distribution, and this is likely to reduce CVD risk.
- Intense endurance training has a highly significant salutary effect on fibrinogen levels in healthy older men.
- Exercise helps in the prevention and treatment of osteoporosis and certain neoplastic diseases, notably colon cancers.
- Exercise reduces manifestations of CHD.
- Exercise improves various indexes of psychological function.
- Exercise reduces depression.
- Exercise improves self-confidence and self-esteem.
- Exercise reduces cardiovascular and neurohumoral responses to mental stress and reduces some type A behavior.

SMOKING

Smoking is the first-degree risk factor for CHD, independent of any other risk factor. It is responsible for approximately 20% of deaths from CHD in men and 17% of deaths in women. Smokers are also between two and four times more likely to suffer from sudden cardiac death. In fact, the risk of CHD is directly proportional to the number of cigarettes smoked per day and the duration of

TABLE 1.5. Examples of common physical activities for healthy adults, by intensity of effort required

Activity	Light <3 METs or <4 kcal/min	Moderate 3–6 METs or 4–6 kcal/min	Vigorous >6 METs or 7 kcal/min
Walking	Walk pacing, normal walk	Briskly, striding, stair walking	Briskly uphill, running, jogging
Cycling	Very light effort	5–9 mph, level terrain or with a few hills	Fast (>10 mph), steep hill terrain
Swimming	Slow treading	Laps for 20 minutes	Lap swimming more than 20 minutes
Conditioning exercise	Light stretching, warming up	Gymnastic exercise, yoga, weight training	Fitness machines, circuit weight training
Sports	Golf powered care	Table tennis, doubles lawn tennis, light badminton, volleyball, golfing, softball, baseball	Singles tennis, squash, intense badminton, soccer, field hockey, ice hockey, lacrosse, basketball, cross-country skiing
Boating	Power boating	Leisurely canoeing	Canoeing rapidly, rowing
Home care	Light house work, dusting	General maintenance	Moving or pushing furniture, digging, masonry
Mowing lawn	Riding mower	Power mower	Hand mower

One MET is equivalent to using one kcal/kg/hour of energy.
Data from Ainsworth BE, Haskell WL, Leon AS, et al. Compendium of physical activities. Med Sci Sports Exerc 1993;25:71–80 Leon AS, Physical fitness In: Wynder EL, ed American Health Foundation, The Book of Health. New York, NY; Franklin Watts; 1981:293 McCardle WD, Katch FI, Katch VL. Exercise Physiology: Energy Nutrition Performance. 2nd Ed. Philadelphia, PA: Lea & Febger; 1986:642.

smoking. Smoking one to four cigarettes a day increases the risk of CHD by two, whereas the risk increases 11 times by smoking over 45 cigarettes a day. A smoker with high blood pressure, high cholesterol, or any other risk factor is more prone to suffer from CHD compared to a nonsmoker. Stopping smoking reduces the risk gradually. Smoking cessation even after the development of CHD is proven to be beneficial. For CHD, the risk of coronary events declines to half within a year and in 10 years it declines to that of person who has never smoked. The risk of stroke declines more slowly. Smoking cessation was associated with a reduction in cardiac event rates of 7% to 47% in three randomized smoking cessation trials that were performed in a primary prevention setting.[27]

Q: What drug therapies are indicated in smoking cessation?

Smoking cessation intervention is a cost-effective way of reducing ill health and prolonging life. Behavioral support and advice from a smoking cessation specialist is helpful in quitting smoking. Taylor and coworkers[29] have shown that 32% of patients will stop smoking at the time of cardiac event and this rate can be significantly increased to 61% by a nurse-managed smoking cessation program.[28] Advice about smoking cessation should include a discussion of nicotine replacement therapy and bupropion, which are effective aids for those smoking more than 10 cigarettes a day. Bupropion has been used in the treatment of depression, but its mode of action in smoking cessation is not clear. However, nicotine replacement therapy is regarded as the pharmacological treatment of choice.

Nicotine replacement therapy or bupropion should be prescribed only for a smoker who commits to a target stop date. The smoker should be offered advice and encouragement to aid smoking cessation. Therapy to aid smoking cessation is chosen according to the smoker's likely compliance, availability of counseling and support, previous experience of smoking cessation aids, contraindications and adverse effects of the products, and the smoker's preferences.

Nicotine Replacement Therapy

Nicotine is available as patches, inhalers, microtabs, nasal spray, gum, and lozenges. Nicotine patches may be used to stop smoking, and their use can double the success rate but only when accompanied by regular counseling. Heart attacks have been reported in users of nicotine patch who continued to smoke. Therefore, smoking must be stopped while using nicotine patches. The patches also are contraindicated in those who previously suffered MI, unstable angina, arrhythmia, or stroke, and during pregnancy and lactation. Three brands of nicotine patches are licensed in the U.K. and two in US:

1. Nicotrol/Nicorette Patch (Pharmacia & Upjohn), 5, 10, 15 mg released over 16 hours
2. Nicotine TTS in the U.K. (Novartis Consumer), 7, 14, 21 mg released over 24 hours
3. Nicoderm CQ/Niquitin CQ (Glaxo SmithKline), 7, 14, 21 mg released over 24 hours

Bupropion

Bupropion was originally researched as an antidepressant drug. It is used in the dosage of 150 mg daily for 6 days, and then 150 mg twice a day; the maximum period of treatment is 7 to 9 weeks. It should be discontinued if abstinence is not achieved at 7 weeks. Elderly patients should be prescribed 150 mg a day maximum. Bupropion may impair driving skills. It is contraindicated in patients with a history of fits, eating disorders, or a brain tumor, or in patients who are experiencing acute symptoms of alcohol or benzodiazepine withdrawal.

References

1. British Heart Foundation. Coronary Heart Disease Statistics, 2003. www.heartstats.org//datapage.asp?id=1652.
2. Ornish D, Brown SE, Scherwitz LW, et al. Can lifestyle changes reverse coronary heart disease? The Lifestyle Heart Trial. Lancet 1990;336: 129–133.
3. Connor WE. Importance of omega-3 fatty acids in health and disease. Am J Clin Nutir 2000; 71(1 suppl):171S–175S.
4. United States Department of Agriculture. Nutrient Data Lab. www. nal.usda.gov/fnic/foodcomp (accessed 1.22.05).
5. GISSI-Prevenzione Investigators. Dietary supplementation with n-3 polyunsaturated fatty acids and vitamin E after myocardial infarction: results of the (GISSI-Prevenzione Trial). Lancet 1999;354:447–455.
6. Burr ML, Fehily MA, Gilber JE, et al. Effects of changes in fat, fish and fiber intakes on death and MI: Diet & Reinfarction Trial (DART). Lancet 1989;2:757–761.
7. Albert CM, Campos H, Stampfer MJ, et al. Blood levels of long chain and n-3 fatty acids and the risk of sudden death. N Engl J Med 2002; 346:1113–1118.
8. Hu FB, Bronner L, Willett WC, et al. Fish and omega-3 fatty acid intake and linolenic acid-rich diet in secondary prevention of CHD. Lancet 1994;343:1454–1459.
9. ATP III Final report. Adopting life-style habits to lower LDL-C and reduce CHD risk. Circulation 2002;106:3253–3280.

10. De Lorgeril M, Salen P, Martin JL, et al. Mediterranean diet, traditional risk factors, and the rate of cardiovascular complications after myocardial infarction: final report of the Lyon Diet Heart Study. Circulation: 1999;99:779–785.

11. Chrysohoou C, Panagiotakos DB, Pistaros C, et al. Adherence to the Mediterranean diet attenuates an inflammation and coagulation process in healthy adults. J Am Coll Cardiol 2004;45:152–158.

12. Mozaffarian D, Ascherio A, Hu F. Interplay between different polyunsaturated fatty acids and risk of CHD in men. Circulation 2005; 111:157–164.

13. Singh RB, Ziaz MA, Sharma JP, et al. Randomised double-blind, placebo-controlled trial of fish oil and mustard oil in patients with suspected acute myocardial infarction: the Indian Experiment of Infarct Survival–4. Cardiovasc Drugs Ther 1997;11:485–491.

14. Thun MJ, Peto R, Lopez AD, et al. Alcohol comsumption and mortality among middle-aged and elderly US adults. N Engl J Med 1997; 337:1705–1714.

15. Maclure M. Demonstraion of deductive meta-analysis: ethanol intake and risk of myocardial infarction. Epidemiol Rev 1993;15:328–351.

16. Beckemeier ME, Bora PS. Fatty acid ethyl esters; potentially toxic products of myocardium ethanol metabolism. J Mol Cell Cardiol 1998; 30:2487–2494.

17. Mukamal KJ, Congrave KM, Mittleman MA, et al. Roles of drinking pattern and types of alcohol consumed in coronary heart disease in men.. N Engl J Med 2003;342(2):109–118.

18. Gorinstein S, Zemser M, Lichman I, et al. Moderate beer consumption and the blood coagulation in patients with coronary artery disease. J Intern Med 1997;241:47–51.

19. Rimm EB, Klatsky A, Grobbee D, et al. Review of moderate alcohol consumption and reduced risk of coronary heart disease: is the effect due to beer, wine, or spirits? BMJ 1996;312:731–736.

20. Blackburn H, Leon AS. Preventive cardiology in practice. Minnestota studies on risk factors reduction. In: Pollock MK, Schmidt DH, eds. Heart Diseases and Rehabilitation, 2nd ed. New York: John Wiley, 1986: 265–301.

21. Greenfield JR, Samaras K, Jenkins AB. Obesity is an important determinant of baseline CRP in monozygotic twins, independent of genetic influences. Circulation 2004;109:3022–3028.

22. Mason J, Colditz G, Stampfer M, et al. A prospective study of obesity and the risk of CAD in women. N Engl J Med 1990;322(13):882–889.

23. Jung R. Obesity as a disease. Br Med Bull 1997;53(2):307–321.

24. Tanasescu M, Leitzmann MF, Rimm EB, et al. Exercise type and intensity in relation to coronary heart disease in men. JAMA 2002; 288(16):23–30.

25. Thompson PD, Buchner D, Ileana CP, et al. Exercise and physical activity in the prevention and treatment of atherosclerotic CVD. Circulation 2003;107:3109–3116.

26. Fletcher G, Balady G, Balirs N, et al. Statement on exercise: benefits and recommendations for physical program for all Americans. Circulation 1996;94:857–862.
27. Gibbons RJ, Chatterjee K, Daley J, et al. ACC/AHA/ACP Guidelines for the management of patients with chronic stable angina. Circulation 1999;99:2829–2848.

Chapter 2
Lipids

Hypercholestrolemia and hypertriglyceridemia are both risk factors for coronary heart disease (CHD) and cardiovascular disease (CVD). Although the association between low-density lipoprotein (LDL) cholesterol and CHD risk is continuous, it is not linear. The risk of CHD rises more steeply with increasing LDL-C level. This results in a curvilinear, or log-linear, association. In other words, when the association between LDL-C and CHD risk is plotted on a log scale, the association becomes linear. The data suggests that for every 30 mg/dL (0.8 mmol) change in LDL-C, the relative risk for CHD is changed in proportion by approximately 30%.[1]

LIPIDS AND LIPOPROTEINS

Q: What are lipids and lipoproteins?
Simple lipids in the body are cholesterol and fatty acids, whereas the complex lipids are cholesterol esters and glycerol esters. Cholesterol is a precursor of bile acids and steroid hormone. Cholesterol esters are produced with the combination of cholesterol and fatty acids, whereas glycerol esters comprise triglycerides and phospholipids. Triglycerides are produced by a combination of glycerol with three units of fatty acid. They are stored in the fatty tissues and act as an important source of energy. Triglycerides are derived from the diet and are also synthesized by the liver. The daily intake of triglyceride is 70 to 150 g. Triglycerides are carried in the body as chylomicrons and are rapidly cleared from the blood to be used as an important source of energy. Some triglycerides are deposited as fat in the body. Phospholipids are formed with a combination of glycerol with a phosphate-containing molecule, rather than fatty acid. Lipids include cholesterol, free fatty acids, triglycerides, and phospholipids.

Cholesterol is a key structural component of cell membrane and is responsible for the synthesis of many other steroids including bile salts, steroid hormones, and vitamin D. Therefore, dietary cholesterol is essential for the body. Dietary intake of cholesterol is 300 to 400 mg daily, and the rest is synthesized in the liver (900 mg/d). Cholesterol and bile acids are secreted into the bile, which passes into the intestine where 50% of cholesterol and 97% of bile acids are reabsorbed and returned to the liver. The units used for cholesterol and triglycerides are either mg/dL or mmol/L. The conversion factors for these calculations are as follows:

Cholesterol: mg/dL = mmol/L × 38.67
Triglycerides: mg/dL = mmol/L × 88.57

Free fatty acids participate in various metabolic processes to produce energy. In the blood these fatty acids are transported, bound to albumin. After absorption, cholesterol, triglycerides, phospholipids, and free fatty acids combine with proteins (called apolipoproteins) to form lipoproteins, which act as a transport vehicle, the aim of which is to deliver lipids to different parts of the body. These contain cholesterol, triglyceride, phospholipids, and protein in various different proportions. High-density lipoproteins contain more protein than lipids.

Three major classes of lipoproteins in a fasting person are low-density lipoproteins (LDLs), high-density lipoproteins (HDLs), and very low density lipoproteins (VLDLs). Intermediate-density lipoproteins (IDLs) are found between VLDL and LDL. LDL-C constitutes 60% to 70% of total cholesterol. It contains lipoprotein B-100 (apo B). HDL cholesterol makes up 20% to 30% of total cholesterol. HDL is subdivided into A-1 and A-11. There is increasing evidence that Lp A-1 containing particles predominate in HDL-2, and are of particular importance in protecting against CHD. VLDL is triglyceride-rich lipoprotein and constitutes 10% to 15% of total cholesterol. The major apolipoproteins of VLDL are apo-100, apo CS (C-1, C-11, C-111), and apo E. VLDL is synthesized in the liver and is a precursor of LDL. Some forms of VLDL, such as VLDL remnants, are more atherogenic, similar to LDL. A fourth lipoprotein is chylomicrons.

Cholesterol is transported in lipoprotein mainly as LDL cholesterol. It is thought that cholesterol is cleared from the arterial wall and carried back to the liver by HDL cholesterol, so-called reverse transport. Chylomicrons are the first lipoproteins to be formed. They transport triglycerides from the intestine to the blood, which delivers triglycerides to the tissues where they are broken down into fatty acids. After chylomicrons have performed this function, the liver absorbs them. Chylomicrons appear in the blood for only 12 hours after a meal. Therefore, the blood test for triglycerides should be done after the patient has fasted for at least 12 hours. The liver synthesizes mainly VLDL, which carries nondietary triglycerides in the blood. Intermediate-density lipoproteins (IDL) or VLDL remnants are formed during conversion of VLDL to LDL. Most of IDL is converted to LDL. The remainder is removed from the blood by the receptors in the liver.

Atherogenic Dyslipidemia

Atherogenic dyslipidemia is a triad of elevated triglycerides, raised small LDL particles, and reduced HDL-C, and it is a risk factor for premature CHD. Typical patients have central obesity and insulin resistance and are physically inactive. Some patients with type 2 diabetes have atherogenic dyslipidemia. The management of atherogenic dyslipidemia includes weight reduction in overweight patients and increased physical activity. Fibrates and nicotinic acid particularly improve all the constituents of this lipid triad.

Non-HDL Cholesterol

Non-HDL cholesterol includes all the lipoproteins that contain apo B, which is a major apolipoprotein of all athrogenic lipoproteins. Its measurement can be used to facilitate risk prediction in patients whose serum triglycerides are high. The Lipid Research Clinic Cohort study showed a stronger correlation with coronary mortality for non–HDL-C than for LDL-C.[2] When the patient has high triglycerides (≥200 mg/dL [2.26 mmol/L]) non–HDL-C better represents the concentration of all atherogenic lipoproteins than LDL-C alone. If triglycerides are >500 mg/dL (5.65 mmol/L), then they do not reliably predict CHD risk.

Total cholesterol (TC) = LDL + VLDL + HDL
Total cholesterol – HDL = LDL + VLDL = non-HDL

Q: What are the causes of primary and secondary dyslipidemia?
Important familial lipid disorders include familial hypercholesterolemia, combined hyperlipidemia, and polygenic hypercholesterolemia. The genetic role in their pathogenesis is discussed in Chapter 6.

Familial Hypercholesteremia (WHO Type IIa)

Familial hypercholesteremia (FH) has a strong association with premature atherosclerosis. The estimated prevalence of the heterozygous type is one in 500 in the general population, whereas the homozygous type is extremely rare, one in a million, and the disease is more severe. The primary genetic defect is an autosomal-dominant disorder in which a mutation is passed from a parent to roughly half the children. The defect leads to the production of a poorly functioning LDL receptor, LDL production is increased, and typically there are tendinous xanthomas, arcus and xanthelasma. The cholesterol level is about 345 mg/dL (9.0 mmol/L). Untreated, the majority of male heterozygotes and half of the female heterozygotes will have a clinical CHD before the age of 60 years. Overall, the mutation detection rate is about 75% in childprobands. To date, more than 400 different mutations causing hypercholesteremia have been reported worldwide.

Familial Combined Hyperlipidemia

Familial combined hyperlipidemia (FCH) is the commonest type of hyperlipidemia in the general population. One in 200 people in the United Kingdom have this disorder. It is characterized by a large number of dense LDLs, causing elevated levels of both cholesterol and triglycerides. The presentation may vary within families with severe Fredrickson phenotypes (IIa, IIb, IV). There is an increased risk for premature atherosclerosis but there are no tendinous xanthomas. Clinically, FCH may simulate FH. The underlying defect is the overproduction of Apo-B-100. The genetics of this disorder are not straightforward, and to date none of the genetic causes have been identified with certainty. Obesity and insulin resistance appear to be common in FCH.

Polygenic Hypercholesterolemia (WHO Type IIa)

Polygenic hypercholesterolemia reflects the interaction of multiple genes and environmental factors such as diet. No particular gene defect is responsible. It is associated with premature CHD. About 7% of first-degree relatives of patients have elevated LDL-C levels.

Primary Isolated Hypertriglyceridemia

This condition is due to excess VLDL in fasting plasma, which is responsible for the patient's turbid appearance. Many patients have a demonstrable secondary cause such as metabolic syndrome. In some patients the disease appears to be familial and with a dominant inheritance. These patients have either World Health Organization (WHO) type IV or V. The extent to which this condition increases the risk of CHD is uncertain.

Causes of Secondary Hyperlipidemia

Certain diseases can increase the level of lipids in the blood despite normal dietary intake. Secondary hyperlipidemia makes up 40% of all hyperlipidemia. The important causes of secondary hyperlipidemia include diabetes, hypothyroidism, chronic renal failure, obstructive liver disease, and drugs that increase LDL cholesterol, such as progestins, anabolic steroids, and corticosteroids. Excessive alcohol intake can increase the triglyceride level. Treating the underlying cause can be successful.

Q: What are the causes of low HDL and what is its management?

Low HDL (<40 mg/dL [1.0 mmol/L]) is an independent risk factor. The causes of low HDL include insulin resistance, cigarette smoking, high carbohydrate diet (>60% of calories), and drugs such as beta-blockers, anabolic steroids, and progestational agents. Other causes include hypertriglyceridemia, being overweight, physical inactivity, type 2 diabetes, and genetic factors.

Management of low HDL includes therapeutic lifestyle changes such as exercise, smoking cessation, weight loss, and reduction of saturated fat and cholesterol in the diet. Raising HDL levels reduces risk, but the current drugs do not raise HDL sufficiently. The advice therefore is to target LDL first. However, if there is low HDL level (with triglycerides ≥200 mg/dL [2.26 mmol]), fibrates or nicotinic acid should be used.

Q: Who should be screened for elevated lipids?

In the absence of current CHD, cholesterol should be tested in patients under 45 years of age as a part of primary prevention if they have any of the following:

- A history of familial hyperlipidemia.
- A personal history of CHD, peripheral vascular disease (PVD), or cardiovascular accidents (CVA).
- A family history of CHD, PVD (especially before the age of 55 years), or hyperlipidemia.
- Diabetes mellitus.
- Hypertension.
- Obesity.
- Chronic renal failure.
- Cigarette smoking.
- Physical stigmata of hyperlipidemia.

In patients 45 years of age or older, the following criteria warrant testing the cholesterol level:

- Men aged 45 to 54 years with two or more cardiovascular (CV) risk factors, and men aged 55 to 64 years with one or more CV risk factors.
- Women aged 55 to 64 years with two or more CV risk factors.

MANAGEMENT

Q: What is the role of exercise and dietary advice in hyperlipidemia?
The essential features of lifestyle changes are weight reduction, increased physical activity, and dietary modifications, such as increased intake of plant stanol/sterol (2 g/d) and increased intake of viscous (soluble) fiber (10–20 g/d). Five to 10 g of viscous fiber per day reduces LDL-C by approximately 15%. Dietary-rich sources of cholesterol are egg yolk, offal, fish, meat, poultry (with skin), butter, and other dairy products. A Total Lifestyle Changes (TLC) diet should be adhered to.

A higher intake of total fat, mostly in the form of unsaturated fat, can help to reduce triglycerides and raise HDL cholesterol in a person with metabolic syndrome. Rigorous dieting can reduce cholesterol by 11 to 22 mg/dL (0.3–0.6 mmol/L). In the Scandinavian trial, although the placebo group was given advice on dietary modification, the run-in levels of cholesterol prior to the initiation of randomized therapy showed no difference over several months, and continued without any real change in patients randomized to the placebo.[3] Various soluble fibers reduce total and LDL-C by similar amounts. Increasing soluble fiber can make a small contribution to dietary therapy to lower cholesterol. The few randomized controlled trials that are available have failed to establish that garlic reduces LDL.

Plant Sterols (Stanol/Sterol Ester)
Sterols are produced in both animals and plants. They are essential components of cell membranes. Cholesterol is an animal sterol. There are about 40 plant sterols, such as beta-sitosterol, campesterol, and stigmasterol. Plant sterols are formed when the delta-5 double bond of the sterol ring of plant is hydrogenated. They can be unsaturated or saturated. Plant sterols are generally ingested from edible vegetable oils (sunflower, rapeseed, soya, maize, and sesame), and are also present in legumes. Bread and cereals, although not a rich source, provide 17% of dietary plant sterol. The average intake in the U.K. is 200 mg per day. Vegetarians consume about 600 to 800 mg daily. Plant stanols and sterols, approximately 2 g per day, can reduce LDL-C by 10% to 15%. The effect of plant

sterol and statins is additive. Some spreads, fortified with plant sterols, such as Benecol in Finland, Flora Proactive in Europe, and Take Control in the United States, are available in retail stores. Until more is known about their side effects, their use should be restricted to those requiring the lowering of cholesterol.

Q: What is the pharmacological treatment for hyperlipidemia?
Drug treatment is divided into those drugs that exert primary effect on total and LDL-cholesterol and those that act on triglycerides. Statins are the drug of choice for lowering cholesterol, but they also reduce triglycerides to some extent. Reduction of the LDL-C level can lower CHD by one third. The following drugs are used for lowering lipids (Table 2.1).

CHOLESTEROL-LOWERING DRUGS

HMG-CoA Reductase Inhibitors
Statins act as specific inhibitors of 3-hydroxyl-3-methyl glutaryl co-enzyme A (HMG-CoA) reductase, the rate-limiting enzyme. They act by blocking the endogenous synthesis of cholesterol through the competitive inhibition of the rate-limiting enzyme responsible for hepatic synthesis of cholesterol. As endogenous synthesis is prevented, the cholesterol requirement of the hepatocyte is met by the uptake of circulating cholesterol via a catabolic LDL receptor on the cell surface. Statins are the most potent compound for reducing the plasma LDL-C level. From the safety point of view, all statins appear similar. Statins, except atorvastatin, are dosed at night because of higher nocturnal cholesterol synthesis. They also moderately increase HDL-C and moderately reduce plasma triglycerides. Pravastatin and rosuvastatin are hydrophilic. Simvastatin lowers C-reactive protein (CRP) by 14 days, independent of its effect on LDH cholesterol.[4] The overall clinical benefits of statins appear greater than would be expected from their effects on LDL-C alone. Important pleiotropic effects[5] of statins in relation to atherogenesis are as follows:

- Improving arterial endothelial function, partly by lowering LDL-C.
- Stabilizing atherosclerotic plaques.
- Decreasing oxidative stress and vascular inflammation.
- Directly enhancing constitutive endothelial nitric oxide synthase (eNOS) activity, thereby increasing the bioavailability of nitric oxide (NO).

TABLE 2.1. Lipid-lowering drugs

Generic name	Daily dose	Comments
Cholesterol-lowering drugs		
HMG CoA reductase inhibitors		*Side-effects*: myopathy especially when used with fibrates, elevated liver transaminase. *Contraindications*: Absolute—acute liver disease; Relative—concomitant use of cyclosporine, antifungal, macrolindes. *Caution* with fibrates, nicotinic acid
Atorvastatin	10–80 mg	
Fluvastatin	20–40 mg	
Pravastatin	10–40 mg	
Simvastatin	10–40 mg	
Rosuvastatin	10–40 mg	
Lovastatin (not in U.K.)	10–80 mg	
Bile-acid sequestrants		*Side-effects*: GIT complaints, decreased absorption of other drugs. *Contraindications*: absolute—familial dysbetalipoproteinemia, triglyceride >400 mg/dL (4.52 mmol/L). Relative—if triglyceride >200 mg/dL/2.26 mmol/d
Cholestyramine	4–16 g	
Colestipol	5–20 g	
Colesevelam (not in U.K.)	2.6–3.8 g	
Cholesterol absorption inhibitor		
Ezetimibe	10 mg	Avoid with hepatic insufficiency

Triglyceride-lowering drugs

Fibrates

Gemfibrozil	600 mg bid	*Side-effects*: myopathy, rhabdomyolysis if used with statins especially gemfibrozil; GIT upset, gall stones. *Contraindications*: severe renal & hepatic disease. *Caution*: monitor creatine kinase levels
Fenofibrate	200 mg	
Bezafibrate m/r	400 mg tid	
Ciprofibrate	100 mg	

Nicotinic acid & its derivative

Nicotinic acid (Niacin)	1–2 g	*Side-effects*: raised blood sugar or uric acid. *Contraindications*: chronic liver disease, gout. Relative—type 2 diabetes
Acipimox	250 mg tid	
Nicotinic acid crystalline	1.5–3 g	
Nicotinic acid extended release	1–2 g	
Nicotinic acid sustained release	1–2 g	

Omega-3 marine derivatives — Refer to pharmaceutical preparations

Statins: LDL ↓ 18–55%, HDL ↑ 5–15%, triglycerides ↓ 7–30%.
Bile acid sequestrant: LDL ↓ 15–30%, HDL ↑ 3–5%, Triglycerides no effect.
Fibrates: LDL ↓ 5–20%, HDL ↑ 10–35%, Triglycerides ↓ 20–50%.
Nicotinic acid: LDL - ↓ 5–25%, HDL - ↑ 15–35%, triglycerides - ↓ 20–50%.

- Modulating membrane microdomain formation, resulting in reduced expression of proteins that specifically inhibit eNOS activation.
- Reducing sterol biosynthesis, thus interfering with the formation of the pathological microdomain, including cholesterol crystalline structures.

Statins directly effect NO, reduce vascular smooth muscle cell proliferation, and reduce the inflammatory cell content of plaque lesions and CRP level in the blood. Lipoproteins or their derivatives can promote local inflammation and thrombogenicity in the arterial wall, and lipid lowering in this context constitutes a form of anti-inflammatory and antithrombotic therapy.[6] The efficacy of statins can be observed in 3 to 4 weeks, so that titration of the dose can be achieved quickly. The reduction of LDL-C is 30% to 35% when equivalent doses of statins are used. The daily doses of statins that have been shown to reduce LDL-C by 30% to 40% are atorvastatin 10 mg, lovastatin 40 mg, pravastatin 40 mg, simvastatin 20 to 40 mg, fluvastatin 40 to 80 mg, and rosuvastatin 5 to 10 mg. When a lipid-lowering therapy is prescribed in high-risk or moderately high-risk patients, the dose of drug should be high enough to achieve 30% to 40% reduction in LDL-C, regardless of baseline LDL-C.

The side effects of statins are uncommon but include minor gastrointestinal disturbances, headache, rash, raised liver enzymes, and raised levels of muscle enzymes. It is recommended that alanine aminotransferase (ALT), formerly SGPT, and aspartate aminotransferase (AST), formerly SGOT, should be measured initially, approximately 12 weeks after starting therapy, and then annually or more frequently if indicated. If these levels rise and persist at three times the upper limit of normal, then the statins should be discontinued. Evaluate muscle symptoms and creatine kinase (CK) initially and then annually. Measure CK if the patient complains of muscle tenderness or pain. Muscle pain, muscle weakness, and myositis have been reported. Rosuvastatin is the only statin to be used with fenofibrates.

The risk of myopathy is higher if the patient suffers from renal impairment or hypothyroidism, or is taking an immune suppressant (i.e., cyclosporine), a fibrate, or nicotinic acid. Statins when used with fibrates may pose serious risk of myositis, and therefore patients need close supervision. Statins are also best discontinued in severe intercurrent illness to avoid the risk of myopathy, and should not be taken by individuals with liver dysfunction or by alcoholics. Recently it was observed that fenofibrate does not interfere with catabolism of statins, and it is likely that it does not substantially increase the risk for clinical myopathy in patients treated with moderate doses of statins.[7] The combination of a statin with nicotinic acid produces a marked reduction of LDL-C and a striking rise in HDL-C. Although most patients can tolerate nicotinic acid, some cannot. Statins may increase the anticoagulant effect of warfarin, although pravastatin does not. Statins are contraindicated during pregnancy or breast-feeding, or in patients with a history of porphyria, active liver disease, or raised liver enzymes.

Bile Acid Sequestrants (Anion Exchange Resins)

Bile acid sequestrants (resins) have for most patients been replaced by fibrates and statins as first-line agents. Sequestrants act by binding bile acids and by preventing their reabsorption, which promotes conversion of cholesterol (in blood) into bile acid by liver, thus enabling increased removal of LDL from the circulation. Sequestrants may cause nausea, vomiting, constipation, and abdominal discomfort. They may interfere with the absorption of folic acid, thyroxine, digoxin, warfarin, and fibrates. They are contraindicated in patients with biliary obstruction. Cholestyramine is the only commonly used sequestrant.

Ezetimibe

Ezetimibe is a selective intestinal cholesterol absorption inhibitor that blocks the absorption of dietary and biliary cholesterol. It can be used with statins or alone. If more aggressive cholesterol lowering is required, then ezetimibe can be used with statin, which results in an additional 18% reduction over that seen with statin alone. Given that when statin doses are doubled an average 6% further LDL-C reduction is observed, there is room for a low-dose statin/ezetimide combination. Its effects on cardiovascular events are entirely unknown.

TRIGLYCERIDES-LOWERING DRUGS

Fibrates

Fibrates' action is achieved by reduction in the level of triglyceride-rich lipoprotein, VLDL, by stimulating lipoprotein lipase, and probably by decreasing peripheral fat breakdown and fatty acid flux back to the liver. Fibrates possibly also have a weak inhibitory effect on HMG-CoA reductase, increase HDL synthesis (a protective effect), and tend to reduce LDL-cholesterol. They have a greater effect on triglyceride levels than on cholesterol levels, and are indicated for moderate to severe hypertriglyceridemia, in mixed hyperlipidemia where the predominant abnormality is hypertriglyceridemia, and in type III dyslipidemia. Fibrates, however, are not the first-line agents for hypercholesterolemia. They are well tolerated and can be used in combination with anion exchange resins in mixed hyperlipidemia, and with nicotinic acid in severe hypertriglyceridemia. They have a similar side-effect profile to statins, and their contraindications and precautions are also similar. Fibrates can potentiate the action of anticoagulants, and careful monitoring is required. Bezafibrates and fenofibrates increase homocysteine in the blood, whereas gemfibrozil does not. Fibrates reduce the risk of CHD events in patients with high triglycerides and low HDL-C, especially when the patient has diabetes and features of metabolic syndrome. When fibrates are added to statins, it is recommended to reduce the dose of statin by 25% to 50% of the maximum dose to minimize the risk of myopathy. Fibrates should be used with statins only with high-risk patients due to the increased side effects. Fenofibrate may be slightly more effective than gemfibrozil in reducing LDL-C in patients with hypercholesterolemia or mixed hyperlipidemia. Due to the risk of myotoxicity including rhabdomyolysis, the combination of a fibrate, particularly gemfibrozil, with a statin requires extreme caution and monitoring of creatine kinase levels.

Nicotinic Acid Derivatives

Nicotinic acid derivatives inhibit the breakdown of fatty tissue, decreasing the availability of fatty acids to the liver, and reducing the formation of VLDL and triglycerides in the liver. It lowers both LDL-C and triglycerides. Niacin is considered to be the most effective pharmaceutical agent for raising HDL-C (National Cholesterol Education Program [NCEP], Adult Treatment Panel [ATP] 111). In hypertriglyceridemia, the reduction is more marked than when triglyceride is normal. Nicotinic acid is particularly useful in increasing HDL-C levels in hypertriglyceridemic patients and is also highly effective in dysbetalipoproteinemia. Nicotinic acid therapy provides a moderate reduction in CHD risk, either when used alone or in combination with other lipid-lowering drugs. The side effects include flushing, rash, abdominal discomfort, and a tendency to raise uric acid and sugar in blood. Rarely, nicotinic acid impairs liver function. These drugs are contraindicated in pregnancy, breast-feeding, and when there is a history of peptic ulcer. Several studies show the efficacy of nicotinic acid for reduction of CHD risk, both when used alone and in combination with statins. Niacin is also indicated for isolated low HDL. It is recommended to monitor uric acid, fasting blood sugar, and ALT/AST. Measure ALT/AST initially, 6 to 8 weeks after starting therapy, and then annually or more frequently if indicated.

Omega-3 Fatty Acids

Fish-oil preparations rich in omega-3 marine triglycerides are useful in the treatment of severe hypertriglyceridemia but have a limited role. They reduce plasma triglycerides probably by inhibiting VLDL synthesis in the liver. Omega-3 marine triglycerides in conjunction with dietary and other measures are indicated in the reduction of plasma triglycerides in patients judged to be at special risk of ischemic heart disease or pancreatitis. Their side effects include nausea and belching. The following combinations are ideal:

- Safest combination: statins and ezetimide, or statins and omega-3.
- Moderately safe combination: statins and nicotinic acid.
- Least safe combination: statins and fibrates.

Q: Who should be offered treatment for raised lipids? Should raised cholesterol be treated in patients over the age of 70 years as a part of primary prevention?

Absolute risk rises with age because of progressive atherosclerosis. Absolute risk reduction is just as good in older age groups as in other high-risk groups. The Prospective Study of Pravastatin in the Elderly at Risk (**PROSPER**) study supports the use of lipid-lowering drugs beyond 72 years of age.[8,9] This trial examined the efficacy of pravastatin in older men and women with a high risk of developing CVD and stroke (and with baseline LDL-C 150 mg/dL [3.9 mmol/L] to 350 mg/dL [9.1 mmol/L]). Pravastatin reduced LDL-C by 34%. The composite end point (coronary death, nonfatal myocardial infarction [MI], and fatal or nonfatal stroke) was reduced by 15%. Major coronary events (nonfatal MI and CHD death) fell by 19% and CHD mortality by 24%. No reduction in stroke was observed, but transient ischemic attacks (TIAs) fell by 25%. Statins are indicated in elderly with or without CVD.

The decision of whether to treat a patient with raised lipids depends on both the lipid profile and the 10-year risk of CHD. Therefore, the risk of CHD should be calculated in all patients using cardiac risk calculators or tables as a part of primary prevention. It should be noted that the ratio of total cholesterol to HDL cholesterol, is used only for calculating the 10-year risk for CHD, and is no longer used on its own as a treatment threshold for raised lipids.

NATIONAL CHOLESTEROL EDUCATION PROGRAM (U.S.) GUIDELINES[1]

- Lowering LDL-C is the main target; once it is achieved, HDL-C and other nonlipid risk factors should be targeted. Total Lifestyle Changes (TLC) should be the first step and should always be part of drug therapy.
- If there is evidence of CHD or CHD equivalents, do a lipoprotein analysis. The CHD risk equivalents carry a risk for major coronary events equal to that of established CHD (i.e., >20% per year). CHD risk equivalents are:
  1. Other clinical forms of atherosclerotic disease (peripheral vascular disease [PVD]), abdominal aortic aneurysm, and symptomatic carotid artery disease
  2. Diabetes
  3. Multiple risk factors that confer a 10-year risk for CHD >20%
- If there is no evidence of CHD, but there are two or more risk factors of CHD, then the Framingham scoring system should be used to identify those who are at 10-year risk and need treatment.
- It is recommended to do a complete lipoprotein profile (total cholesterol, LDL-C, HDL-C, and triglycerides) as the preferred initial test rather than screening for total cholesterol and HDL-C alone.
- It classified cholesterol levels as follows:
  - LDL-C <100 mg/dL (2.6 mmol/L) optimal; 100–129 mg/dL (2.6–3.4 mmol/L) optimal/above optimal; 130–159 md/dL (3.4–4.2 mmol/L) borderline high; 160–189 mg/dL (4.2–4.9 mmol/L) high; and ≥190 mg/dL (4.9 mmol/L) very high.
  - HDL-C <40 mg/dL (1.0 mmol/L) low and ≥60 (1.6 mmol/L) high.

Three categories of risk that modify the LDL-C goal are identified:

1. High risk includes established CHD and CHD risk equivalents for which the LDL-C goal is <100 mg/dL (2.6 mmol/L) and drug therapy is initiated at >100 mg/dL (2.6 mmol/L).
   - In high-risk patients, the recommended LDL-C goal is <100 mg/dL, but when the risk is very high the LDL-C goal of <70 mg/dL (1.8 mmol/L) is a therapeutic option on the basis of trials.
   - If LDL is ≥100 mg/dL, then a lipid-lowering drug is indicated simultaneously with lifestyle changes.
   - If baseline LDL-C is <100 mg/dL, then initiation of drug therapy to achieve LDL level <70 mg/dL is a therapeutic option.

- If a high-risk patient has elevated triglycerides or low HDL, then fibrate or nicotinic acid could be combined with LDL-lowering drug. If triglyceride is ≥200 mg/dL (2.26 mmoL), then non-HDL is a secondary target for treatment, with a goal of 30 mg/dL (0.8 mmol/L) higher than the identified LDL-C.

2. Moderate risk includes patients with two or more risk factors with a 10-year risk of 10% to 20% for which the LDL-C goal is <130 mg/dL (3.4 mmol/L). This group should be assessed by the Framingham risk scoring into three levels: those with >20% risk, those with 10–20% risk, and those with <10% risk. Patients with >20% risk were classified as high risk; for them the LDL-C goal is <100 mg/dL (2.6 mmol/L). For others with two or more risk factors and a 10-year risk of ≤20%, the LDL-C goal is <130 mg/dL (3.4 mmol/L). If the risk is 10% to 20%, then drug therapy should be considered if the LDL is ≥130 mg/dL (3.4 mmol/L) after a trial of dietary therapy. When the 10-year risk is ≤10%, an LDL-lowering drug can be considered if the LDL is ≥160 mg/dL (4.2 mmol/L) on maximum dietary therapy.

For moderately high-risk patients, the LDL-C goal is <130 mg/dL (3.4 mmol/L), and the LDL goal of <100 mg/dL is a therapeutic option. When LDL is 100 to 129 mg/dL at baseline or on lifestyle measures, initiation of lipid-lowering drugs to achieve an LDL-C of <100 mg/dL is a therapeutic option. In high-risk or moderate-risk patients, the dose of lipid-lowering drugs should be sufficient to achieve at least a 30% to 40% reduction in LDL-C.

3. Mild risk includes at most one risk factor with a 10-year risk less than 10%; then the LDL goal is <160 mg/dL (4.2 mmol/L). For low-risk patients, the LDL goal is <160 mg/dL, and drugs should be initiated at >190 mg/dL (4.9 mmol/L). If the LDL-C is 160 to 189 mg/dL after dietary therapy, drug therapy is optional.

Other Lipid Targets

The non–HDL-C (VLDL + LDL-C) goal is 30 mg/dL higher than the LDL-C goal when triglycerides ≥200 mg/dL (2.26 mol/L). Statins lower non–HDL-C and LDL-C to a similar percentage.

Q: What are the benefits of lipid-lowering drugs in primary prevention?

In primary prevention other risk factors need to be evaluated, because in the absence of other risk factors drug therapy may not be indicated. Absolute CHD risk should be assessed. Additional factors such as family history, genetic hyperlipidemia, renal disease, ethnicity, socioeconomic deprivation, serious comorbidity, and the patient's wishes should also be considered in determining whom to treat. Following are the important studies to support the use of lipid-lowering drugs in primary prevention.

The West of Scotland Coronary Prevention Study (WOSCOPS), a randomized, placebo-controlled, double-blind trial, was a landmark in the evaluation of the benefits of statin therapy.[10,11] This study included 6596 men only, aged 45 to 64 years, with no previous history of heart attack, but some cases of stable angina were included. These subjects had high cholesterol (total cholesterol >250 mg/dL (6.5 mmol/L) and LDL-C was 173 to 230 mg/dL (4.5–6 mmol/L). In this study, pravastatin 40 mg daily was prescribed, and the subjects were followed for 5 years. The study resulted in a fall of total cholesterol by 20%, LDL-C by 26%, and triglycerides by 12%, and HDL-C increased by 5%. It was noted that heart attacks (fatal and nonfatal) were reduced by 31%, and all-cause mortality by 22%. There was no increase in noncardiac death, and benefit was derived by all ages equally. The need for revascularization was also reduced. It was also demonstrated that patients with a greater absolute pretreatment risk of heart attack or angina, including older men (>55 years), smokers, those with an HDL level of <42 mg/dL (1.1 mmol/L), and patients with multiple risk factors, experienced an increased absolute benefit from treatment with statins (pravastatin).

The Air Force Coronary Atherosclerosis Prevention Study (AFCAPS), a randomized trial, was conducted in 5000 men and 1000 women attending an outpatient clinic in Texas.[12] This study compared lovastatin 20 to 40 mg daily [titrated to achieve a target LDL-C of <110 mg/dL (2.84 mmol/L)] or placebo with diet on the incidence of first cardiac event. Patients had an average baseline cholesterol of 220 mg/dL (5.71 mmol/L), HDL-C of 39 mg/dL (0.94 mmol/L) for men and 41 mg/dL (1.03 mmol/L) for women, and an LDL cholesterol of 150 mg/dL (3.88 mmol/L). They had an annual CHD risk of 1.3% (about 13% in 10 years). After 5.2 years of treatment with lovastatin, total cholesterol fell by 18%, LDL-C fell by 25%, triglycerides fell by 15%, and HDL-C increased by 6%. The incidence of acute CHD events (fatal or nonfatal MI, unstable angina, or sudden cardiac death) was reduced by 37% and revascularization by 30%. Total mortality was not affected, but this was not an issue in this study. There was no evidence of an increase in noncardiovascular death.

In the Anglo-Scandinavian Cardiac Outcomes Trial-Lipid Lowering Arm (ASCOT-LLA) study, 19,342 hypertensive patients, 40 to 79 years old and having at least three other cardiovascular risk factors, were randomized to one of two antihypertensive regimens.[13] Among these individuals, 10,305 were in addition randomly assigned atorvastatin 10 mg or placebo. Although the trial was to run for 5 years, it was stopped after 3.3 years because of impressive results. At that point, in the atorvastatin group, the incidence of fatal and nonfatal stroke was reduced by 27%, total cardiovascular (CV) events by 21%, and total coronary events by 29%. There was a non-significant trend toward reduction of total mortality in the atorvastatin group. It was concluded that LDL-C lowering with atorvastatin had considerable potential to reduce the risk for CVD in primary prevention in individuals with multiple cardiovascular risk factors.

Q: What is the evidence that lipid lowering is effective in secondary prevention?

Clinical trials have shown that secondary prevention leads to less progression and more regression of preexisting coronary athero-sclerotic lesions. The Scandinavian Simvastatin Survival Study (4S) was a double-blinded, randomized, placebo-controlled trial.[3] It recruited 4444 men and women aged 35 to 70 years who had a history of heart attack or angina, with a cholesterol level between 210 and 300 mg/dL (5.5–8 mmol/L) and a triglyceride level ≤223 mg/dL (2.5 mmol/L) Half were given simvastatin 20 to 40 mg, and half were given placebo. Both groups were reviewed every 5 years. It was noted that in the simvastatin group, the total cholesterol fell by 25%, LDL-C fell by 35%, triglycerides fell by 10%, and HDL-C increased by 8%. The following results were calculated:

- 30% reduction in total mortality
- 34% reduction in major coronary events, both men and women
- No increase in noncardiac deaths

This study also showed that simvastatin reduced the risk of major coronary events in women to the same extent as in men. Survival rates in those over 60 years of age improved.

The Cholesterol and Recurrent Events Study (CARE), a double-blinded, placebo-controlled, randomized trial, recruited 4159 patients, aged 21 to 75 years, who were 3 to 20 months post-MI.[14] This study has provided a number of new and important insights into the benefits of statin therapy in men and women with "average" total cholesterol (<240 mg/dL [6.2 mmol/L]) who had suf-fered a heart attack. CARE recruited heart attack survivors with this average total cholesterol level. They were treated with pravas-tatin 40 mg daily or placebo. The object of treatment was to assess the effects of pravastatin therapy on rates of nonfatal MI and on CHD deaths in post-MI patients without elevated total cholesterol, who continued to receive other post-MI therapy (i.e., aspirin, beta-blocker, revascularization). The primary outcome was fatal coronary disease or confirmed nonfatal heart attack. Patients were followed for 5 years. Fourteen percent of the patients were women and the average age at entry was 59 years. A good number of these patients underwent various coronary procedures as well as receiving concomitant medication, particularly aspirin. It was found that LDL-C fell by 32%, fatal and nonfatal MI by 24%, stroke by 31%, coronary artery bypass graft (CABG) by 26%, and percutaneous transluminal coronary angioplasty (PTCA) by 22%.

Both these trials (4S and CARE) have shown beyond doubt that statins prevent acute coronary events. These benefits are seen in men and women up to the age of 80 years with total cholesterol level of 155 mg/dL (4.0 mmol/L) and above. There is additional evidence from 4S and CARE that hospitalisation for angina, presumably unstable angina, is reduced. The large statin trials also consistently show that these drugs reduce the need for revascularization procedures.

The Long-Term Intervention with Pravastatin in Ischemic Disease (LIPID) Study recruited 9014 subjects (17% female) in Australia and New Zealand, with an average cholesterol level of 5.65 mmol/L (218 mg/dL), who were randomized to pravastatin 40 mg daily or placebo.[15] After 6 years' follow-up in the group taking pravastatin, total cholesterol fell by 18%, LDL cholesterol fell by 25%, triglycerides fell by 11%, and HDL increased by 5%. The following results were noted:

- All-cause mortality fell by 22%.
- Coronary heart disease deaths fell by 24%.
- Fatal CHD and nonfatal heart attack fell by 24%.
- Total strokes fell by 19%.

The Myocardial Ischemic Reduction with Aggressive Cholesterol Lowering (MIRACL) Study recruited 3086 patients and studied the benefits of giving atorvastatin 80 mg/d within 24 to 96 hours of an acute coronary syndrome.[16] After 16 weeks, it was noted that there was reduction of 16% in deaths, nonfatal heart attack, cardiac arrest, and severe angina requiring hospitalization. The incidence of stroke was significantly reduced in the group using atorvastatin. Atorvastatin therapy reduced the average LDL-C from 123 mg/dL (3.2 mmol/L) at baseline to 72 mg/dL (1.9 mmol/L).

The Provastatin or Atorvastatin Evaluation and Infarction Therapy (PROVE-IT) study was designed to assess whether intensive LDL lowering reduces major coronary events, including mortality, more than "standard" LDL-C lowering with statin therapy in high-risk patients.[17] In this study 2162 patients who were hospitalized for acute coronary syndrome (ACS) within the preceding 10 days were randomized to atorvastatin 80 mg or pravastatin 40 mg. At the end of 2 years, the composite cardiovascular end point (death from any cause, MI, unstable angina, [UA], and stroke) was reduced by 16% with atorvastatin compared to pravastatin. The results of the PROVE-IT trial suggest that more intensive LDL therapy reduces major cardiovascular events with ACS compared with less intensive therapy.

This study is indicative of statin's ability to reduce the development of, progression of, and severity of chronic stable angina and ACS. Lowering cholesterol levels with statins reduces the incidence of fatal and nonfatal strokes and total mortality. Hence, treatment with a statin must be considered for all patients with known coronary disease. The pleiotropic effects of statins are described elsewhere in this chapter.

Q: How low should the cholesterol level be?

There are several ongoing studies looking at this question critically. Reducing the LDL-C by more than 24% as in the WOSCOPS study[9,10] or doubling the statin dose as in the AFCAPS[12] did not result in any further reduction in the coronary event rate. In this context it is important to know that the baseline cholesterol level predicted the coronary risk as opposed to the cholesterol level achieved with treatment.

Recent trials, however, suggest that additional benefits could be gained with a more aggressive approach to cholesterol levels reductions in patients who have undergone a revascularization procedure or who are at high risk. It is suggested that the LDL-C should be reduced to below 95 mg/dL (2.5 mmol/L). Evidence from the Heart Protection Study demonstrated that the lowering of LDL-C from 115 mg/dL (3.0 mmol/L) to 65 mg/dL (1.7 mmol/L) produced a risk reduction of 25%, which was similar to that produced by a 40 mg/dL (1 mmol/L) reduction seen at a higher LDL cholesterol level.[18] The results suggest that reducing serum LDL-C for any baseline further lowers the risk in high-risk patients. The trial did not identify a threshold LDL-C level below which no further reduction in risk occurred. The Post Coronary Artery Bypass Study suggested that only when the LDL-C reduction was >45% did evidence of plaque regression occur. The Reversal of Atherosclerosis with

Aggresive Lipid Lowering (REVERSAL) Trial showed that in patients with CHD, intensive lipid lowering with atorvastatin (80 mg) reduced the risk of coronary atherosclerosis compared with pravastatin (40 mg).[22]

Q: Is a raised level of triglycerides a risk factor? What are its causes and what are the treatment options?

A raised plasma triglyceride concentration (normal <150 mg/dL [1.7 mmol/L]) is a risk factor for fatal and nonfatal cardiovascular events (in particular MI) independent of the levels of LDL-C and/or HDL levels (Prospective Cardiovascular Munster [PROCAM] study[23]). The risk increases in proportion to the rise in the triglyceride level. If very high triglycerides are due exclusively to a catabolic defect of serum triglyceride (e.g., deficiencies of lipoprotein lipase or apo C-11), the individual may not be at increased risk from CHD. A meta-analysis of 17 prospective population-based studies found that hypertriglyceridemia is an independent risk factor for CVD.[19] Another meta-analysis of six cohorts showed that, without adjustment for HDL, for every 82 mg/dL (1 mmol/L) increase in the triglyceride level there was a 76% increased risk of CHD in women and a 32% increased risk in men.[20] When adjusted for HDL, the risk remained significant at 37% and 14%, respectively. Small forms of VLDL, IDL, and LDL-C may rapidly penetrate the endothelium and are highly atherogenic.Triglyceride-rich-remnant lipoprotein data show a direct relationship between (small) LDL/IDL and athrogenesis. Triglyceride-rich lipoprotein comprises many metabolically modified lipoprotein particles. The ability of these particles to enter the subendothelial layer largely depends on their size. Remnant lipoproteins derived from chylomicrons or VLDL (for example, lipoprotein subclasses LP-B: C, LP-B: C: E, and LP-A-11: B: C: D: E) have also been shown to promote athrogenesis.[21] Chylomicrons and very large VLDL particles are unable to pass through the endothelial layer, but smaller VLDL, IDL, and LDL particles can do so.

Athrogenic changes accompanying hypertriglyceridemia are low HDL, raised VLDL, increased small dense LDL-C, postprandial lipidemia, and coagulation changes. The thrombotic effect of hypertriglyceridemia is due to the increased secretion of plasminogen activating inhibitor (PAI) and factor VII. Triglyceride accumulation is not a feature of athlerosclerotic plaque, but triglyceride-rich lipoprotein also contains cholesterol esters, and it is likely that some of these are directly athrogenic. The concentration of remnant particles associated with apo C-111 is related more to the development of atherosclerosis than are triglycerides per se.

Zilversmit was the first to report that triglyceride-rich lipoprotein might be atherogenic and that the degree of postprandial lipoprotein metabolism may play an important role in atherogenesis.[24] Triglyceride-rich lipoprotein is VLDL (remnant lipoprotein), which is equal to TC-HDL.

In the Monitored Atherosclerosis Regression Study (MARS), triglyceride-rich proteins were particularly correlated with the rate of progression of mild to moderate (<50% stenosis) rather than severe (≥50% stenosis) coronary lesions[25]. VLDL-C, VLDL-triglyceride, VLDL-apo B, apo C-111, apo E in VLDL + LDL, and apo E in HDL all predicted subsequent coronary events in the CARE study.

High levels of triglycerides usually occur with being overweight, physical inactivity, cigarette smoking, excess alcohol intake, high carbohydrate diet (60% of total calories), medical conditions such as type 2 diabetes, chronic renal failure, nephrotic syndrome, and certain drugs (steroids, retinoids, high doses of beta-blockers) and genetic disorders (familial hyperlipidemia). Clinically, it is observed in patients with the metabolic syndrome. Very high levels may be due to a genetic pattern (i.e., familial types), familial lipoprotein lipase deficiency, or familial apolipoproteins deficiency. Atherogenic remnants can be lowered by weight reduction in overweight individuals and by the use of lipid-lowering drugs (statin, fibrates, and nicotinic acid). Lifestyle modification (e.g., diet, TLC, exercise, reduced alcohol, etc.) should be introduced. Most statins lower triglycerides to some extent. Triglyceride levels are classified as follows:

Normal: <150 mg/dL (1.70 mmol/L)
Borderline: 150–199 mg/dL (1.70–2.26 mmol/L)
High: >200 mg/dL (2.26 mmol/L)

Triglyceride levels should be managed as follows (Adult ATP 111):

- If 150–199 mg/dL (1.7–2.26 mmol/L) or HDL <40 md/dL (1.0 mmol/L), then emphasize weight management, physical activity, and smoking cessation.
- If the triglyceride level is 200 to 499 mg/dL (2.26–5.64 mmol/L), then after LDL-lowering therapy, consider fibrates or niacin.
- If the triglyceride level is ≥500 mg/dL (5.65 mmol/L), then consider fibrates or niacin before LDL-lowering therapy. Also consider omega-3 fatty acids as adjunct therapy.

References

1. Grundy S, Cleeman J, Merz CN, et al. NCEP Report. Implications of recent clinical trials for the National Cholesterol Education Programme, Adult Treatment Panel 111 Guidelines. Circulation 2004; 110:227–239.
2. Cui Y, Blumenthal RS, Flaws JA, et al. Non-HDL-C as a predictor of cardiovascular disease mortality. Arch Intern Med 2001;161:1413–1419.
3. Scandinavian Simvastatin Survival Study Group. Randomized trial of cholesterol lowering in 4444 patients with coronary heart disease. Lancet 1994;344:1383–1389.
4. Plenge JK, Hernandiz TL, et al. Simvastatin lowers CRP within 14 days. Circulation 2002;106(12):1447–1452.
5. Davigan J. Beneficial cardiovascular pleiotropic effects of statin. Circulation 2004;109(suppl iii):39–43.
6. Aikawa M, Voglic SJ, Sugiyama S, et al. Dietary lipid lowering reduces tissue factor expression in rabbit atheroma. Circulation 1999;100: 1215–1222.
7. Prueksaritanoni T, Taug C, Qiu Y, et al. Effects of fibrates on metabolism of statins in human hepatocytes. Drug Metab Dispos 2002;30: 1280–1287.
8. Shepherd J, Blauw GJ, Murphy MB, et al. The design of a prospective study of pravastatin in the elderly at risk (PROSPER). Am J Cardiol 1999;84:1192–1197.
9. Shepherd J, Blauw GJ, Murphy MB, et al. Pravastatin in elderly individuals at risk of vascular disease: a randomized control. Lancet 2002; 360:1623–1630.
10. Shepherd J, Cobbe SM, Ford I, et al, for the West of Scotland Coronary Prevention Study Group. Prevention of CHD with pravastatin in men with hypercholestrolaemia. N Engl J Med 1995;333:1301–1307.
11. West of Scotland Coronary Prevention Study Group. Influence of pravastatin and plasma lipids on clinical events in the West of Scotland Coronary Prevention Study (WOSCOPS). Circulation 1998;97: 1440–1445.
12. Downs JR, Clearfield M, Weis S, et al. Primary prevention of acute coronary events with lovastatin in men and women with cholesterol levels: results of AFCAPS/TEXCAPS Research Group. JAMA 1998;279: 1615–1622.
13. Sever PS, Dahlof B, Poulter, et al. Prevention of coronary and stroke events with atorvastatin in hypertensive patients who have average or lower average than average cholesterol concentration, in the ASCOT-LLA; a multicentre randomized controlled trial. Lancet 2003;362: 1149–1158.
14. Sacks FM, Pfeffer MA, Moye LA, et al. The effects of pravastatin on coronary events after myocardial infarction in patients with average cholesterol levels. N Engl J Med 1996;335:1001–1009.

15. Lipid Study (CARE). Prevention of cardiovascular events and death with pravastatin in patients with coronary heart disease and broad range of cholesterol levels. N Engl J Med 1998;339:1349–1357.
16. Schwartz GG, Olsson AG, Ezekowitz MD, et al. Myocardial ischaemic reduction with aggressive cholesterol lowering (MIRACL). JAMA 2001; 285(13):1711–1718.
17. PROVE-IT (Cannon CP, Braunwald E, McCabe CH, et al. Provastatin or Atorvastatin Evaluation and Infarction Therapy. Intensive vs moderate lipid lowering with statins after acute coronary syndrome. N Engl J Med 2004;350:1495–1505.
18. Heart Protection Study. MRC/BHF Heart Protection Study of cholesterol lowering with simvastatin in 20,536 high-risk individuals: a randomized placebo trial. Lancet 2002;360:7–22.
19. Cullen P. Evidence that triglycerides are an independent CHD risk factor. Am J Cardiol 2000;86:943–949.
20. Hakonon JE, Austin MA. Plasma triglyceride level is a risk factor cardiovascular disease independent of high density lipoprotein cholesterol level: a meta analysis of population-based prospective studies. J Cardiovasc 1996;3:213–219.
21. Fruchart JC, Nierman MC, Stroes ESG, et al. New risk factors for atherosclerotic patient risk assessment. Circulation 2004:109;111–153.
22. Nissen SE, Tuzcu EM, Schoenhagen P, et al. Reversal of Atherosclerosis with Aggressive Lipid Lowering (REVERSAL) Investigators. N Engl J Med 2005;352(1):29–38.
23. Cullen P, Schulte H, Assmann G. Smoking, lipoproteins and coronary heart disease risk. Data from the Munster Heart Study (PROCAM). Eur Heart J 1998;19(11)1632–1641.
24. Couillard C, Bergeron N, Prud'homme D, et al. Postprandial triglyceride response in visceral obesity in men. Diabetes 1998;47(6):953–960.
25. Hodis HN, Mack WJ, Azen SP, et al. Triglyceride- and cholesterol-rich lipoproteins have a differential effect on mild/moderate and severe lesion progression as assessed by quantitative coronary angiography in a controlled trial of lovastatin. Circulation 1994;90(1)42–49.

Chapter 3
Diabetes Mellitus

Some 18.2 million Americans have been diagnosed with diabetes mellitus (type 2 diabetes, 2002 data), and another 5.4 million are estimated to remain undiagnosed. Ninety percent have type 2 diabetes. Data from the World Health Organization (WHO) suggest that in 2000 the global prevalence of diabetes exceeded 176 million; this is projected to increase to over 370 million by 2030.[1] Most of this high prevalence, and the vast majority of the projected increase, is accounted for by type 2 diabetes and is attributed to the global rise of a sedentary lifestyle associated with excess energy intake and obesity. The problem is further compounded due to the fact that type 2 diabetes is increasingly diagnosed in young adults and children. In the United Kingdom Prospective Diabetes Study (UKPDS), the proportion of patients treated with insulin increased from approximately 40% to 70% over 15 years.[2] The increase in mortality and morbidity among people with coronary heart disease (CHD) is related to complications associated with diabetes. The risk of CHD in a diabetic patient is more than doubled with the coexistence of hypertension. In the Multiple Risk Factor Intervention Trial, predictors of cardiovascular disease (CVD) mortality were assessed among men with and without diabetes.[3] The risk of CVD in men with diabetes increased more steeply over a 12-year period than it did in men without diabetes, even after accounting for the presence of other risk factors of CVD. Although generally cardiovascular mortality is greater among men, diabetes is the only disease that causes women to have cardiovascular mortality similar to that of men. A longer duration of diabetes in women was associated with an increase risk of CHD. The Nurses Health Survey showed a strong positive association between type 2 diabetes and CHD, ischemic stroke, and cardiovascular mortality. The Framingham data show that most men with diabetes have 10-year risk of CHD >20%; in control women, however, the risk rarely exceeded the 20% level.

DIAGNOSIS AND ASSESSMENT

Q: What are the diagnostic criteria for the diagnosis of diabetes?
Diabetes is a group of metabolic diseases characterized by hyper-glycemia resulting from defects in insulin secretion, insulin action or both. The classifications of the American Diabetes Association (ADA) and WHO are very similar (Table 3.1).

Q: How does the metabolic syndrome increase the risk of CHD and how should it be managed?
On the basis of data from the Third National Health and Nutrition Examination Survey, about 25% of adult Americans suffer from the metabolic syndrome, and these individuals are at increased risk of CVD. In the Framingham study, the metabolic syndrome alone pre-dicted 25% of all new-onset CVD. The 10-year risk in men with the metabolic syndrome but without diabetes generally ranges from 10% to 20%; fewer women were detected in the 8-year follow up, and probably most were under 50 years of age. Standardized mor-tality rates for CHD in the U.K. are increased by approximately 40% among South Asians immigrants, an increase that is attribut-able to a combination of metabolic variables, which constitutes the insulin syndrome (syndrome X, metabolic syndrome, and Raven's syndrome) (Table 3.2).[4] The metabolic syndrome consists of a variety of cardiovascular risk factors. Different organizations use slightly different criteria for its diagnosis. Adult Treatment Panel (ATP) 111 uses the term *metabolic syndrome* to avoid the implica-tion that insulin resistance is the primary or only cause of associ-ated risk factors.

South Asians develop insulin resistance whenever mildly or moderately overweight. This population can be said to have

TABLE 3.1. Diagnostic criteria of diabetes mellitus

Blood glucose status	Plasma glucose level
Diabetes mellitus	
Fasting glucose, or	≥126 mg/dL (7.0 mmol/L)
2-hr postglucose load, or	≥200 mg/dL (11.1 mmol/L)
Both	
Impaired glucose tolerance	
Fasting (if measured), and	<126 mg/dL (7.0 mmol/L)
2-hr postglucose load	140–200 mg/dL (7.8–11.1 mmol/L)
Impaired fasting glucose (IFG)	
Fasting glucose, and	110–126 mg/dL (6.1–7.0 mmol/L)
if measured, 2-hr post-glucose load	<140 mg/dL (7.8 mmol/L)

TABLE 3.2. Diagnostic criteria of the metabolic syndrome

World Health Organization (WHO)

Insulin resistance, identified by one of the following:
  Type 2 diabetes
  Impaired fasting glucose
  Impaired glucose tolerance
Plus any two of the following:
  BP ≥140 systolic or ≥90 diastolic or antihypertensive medication
  Triglycerides ≥150 mg/dL (1.7 mmol/L)
  HDL-C, in men <35 mg/dL (0.9 mmol/L), in women <39 mg/dL
    (1.0 mmol/L)
  BMI >30 kg/m^2/or waist/hip ratio in men >0.9, in women >0.85
  Urinary albumin excretion rate ≥20 µg/min or creatinine ratio ≥30 mg/g

National Cholesterol Education Program (NCEP) Adult Treatment Panel III

Concomitant presence of three or more of the following:
  Impaired fasting glucose
  High blood pressure ≥130/≥85 mm Hg
  Elevated triglycerides ≥150 mg/dL (≥1.7 mmol/L)
  HDL-C, in men <40 mg/dL (<1.03 mmol/L), in women <50 mg/dL
    (<1.29 mmol/L)
  Waist circumference, in men >40 inches (>102 cm), in women
    >35 inches (>88 cm)

primary insulin resistance. Weight gain, however, increases primary insulin resistance. Insulin resistance is present not only in type 2 diabetes but also to a lesser degree among the majority of overweight people with normal glucose tolerance. Most people with categorical obesity (body mass index [BMI] ≥30 kg/m^2] have postprandial hyperinsulinemia and relatively low insulin sensitivity, but variation in insulin sensitivity exists even within the obese population. It also exists in 25% of nonobese persons with normal glucose tolerance. There is some evidence that some part of insulin resistance is inherited, and it may increase the risk of type 2 diabetes in other family members.

Insulin resistance can be defined as a condition in which a normal amount of insulin produces a less than normal biological response; as a result a state of hyperinsulinism is produced. Hyperinsulinism is a risk factor for CVD. It has been demonstrated that insulin can produce changes in vascular tissue consistent with atherosclerosis. It is postulated that hyperinsulinism stimulates endothelial and vascular smooth muscle cell proliferation, by means of the hormone's action on growth factor receptors, subse-

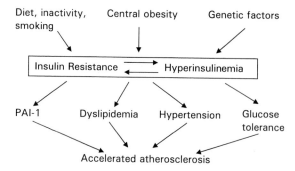

FIGURE 3.1. Relationship between insulin resistance and hyperinsulinemia in cardiovascular risk factors. PAI, plasminogen activator inhibitor.

quently initiating atherosclerosis. The effect of insulin is independent of the effects of cholesterol, blood pressure, body weight, or cigarette smoking. Hypertension and dyslipidemia can occur together in the absence of diabetes but insulin resistance may still be the underlying link. Insulin resistance increases blood pressure by a variety of mechanisms.

Hyperuricemia is a feature of insulin resistance syndrome, although the exact relationship is not clear. Insulin resistance and the resultant hyperinsulinemia are the factors linking hypertension and the metabolic changes (Fig. 3.1). Insulin resistance is also associated with high normal blood pressure. Hyperuricemia is found in about 40% of hypertensive patients, particularly when there is renal impairment. Hyperuricemia correlates with hypertension, glucose intolerance, and dyslipidemia, which are markers for coronary artery disease. Prothrombotic and proinflammatory states (e.g., raised C-reactive protein [CRP]) are characteristic features. Also there are elevated levels of fibrinogen, plasminogen activator inhibitor-1, tissue-type plasminogen activator antigen, factor VII, and factor XII. Patients with the metabolic syndrome are at increased risk of developing premature large-vessel disease (i.e., CHD, stroke, and peripheral vascular disease).

Analysis from the Framingham study has shown that patients with triglyceride levels ≥150 mg/dl (1.70 mmol/L) and high-density lipoprotein (HDL) levels <40 mg/dL (1.0 mmol/L) are characterized by a significantly increased cardiovascular risk. High triglycerides and low HDL-C are an important component of the metabolic syndrome. Leptin is a protein that plays a role in fat metabolism and closely correlates with insulin resistance and other markers of the metabolic syndrome, independent of obesity. Elevated leptin levels are proposed as an independent risk factor for CHD.[5] Hyper-insulinemia increases sodium retention, thereby contributing to or causing hypertension. Ridker et al.[6] advocate adding high-sensitivity CRP (hsCRP) as a clinical criterion for the metabolic syndrome and for the creation of an hsCRP-modified CHD risk score useful for global risk prediction in men and women. The CRP levels correlate with other components of the metabolic syndrome that are not easily measured in clinical practice, including fasting insulin, microalbuminurea, and impaired fibrinolysis. It also predicts type 2 diabetes.

Causes

The main causes of the metabolic syndrome are being overweight, physical inactivity, and genetic factors. Abdominal obesity, atherogenic dyslipidemia, hypertension, insulin resistance with or without glucose intolerance, prothrombotic states, and proinflammatory states characterize it. There are a number of possible mechanisms by which insulin might be causally related to hypertension. These include an effect of insulin on the renin-angiotensin-aldosterone system, sodium absorption in kidneys, sympathetic nervous system activity, and enhanced vascular growth.

Management

Six components of the metabolic syndrome should be addressed:

1. Abdominal obesity: diet, exercise, weight reduction.
2. Atherogenic dyslipidemia: no drug is specifically indicated. Some data suggest that fibrates reduce CVD risk; low-density lipoprotein (LDL)-C target is <100 mg/dL (2.6 mmol/L). For high triglyceride and low HDL, consider fibrates or niacin.
3. Hypertension: see Chapter 4.
4. Insulin resistance with or without glucose intolerance: metformin and thiazolidinediones are useful. Antiplatelet agents such as aspirin reduce insulin resistance, but it is not proven that these agents reduce CHD risk.
5. Proinflammmatory: no specific drug, but aspirin and statins are useful.
6. Prothrombotic state: no specific drug, but antiplatelets and statins are useful.

A drug therapy category of so-called dual peroxisome proliferator-activated receptor (PPAR) agonists is currently under development. These agents target both PPAR-γ and PPAR-α, thereby simultaneously improving insulin resistance, glucose intolerance, elevated triglycerides, and low HDL.

Q: How do diabetic complications predict cardiovascular risk?
Complications of diabetes depend on the duration of diabetes and the degree of its control. A poorly controlled diabetic is more prone to suffer complications. Patients with type 2 diabetes mellitus have a twofold to threefold increased incidence of disease related to atheroma, and those who present in their 40s and 50s have a twofold increased total mortality. Diabetes affects both macro- and microvascular vessels. In the U.K., the incidence of macrovascular complications is twice that of microvascular disease. Diabetic complications are related to increased mortality and morbidity among CHD patients.

Macrovascular Complications
Macrovascular complications include CHD, CVD, (e.g., stroke, transient ischemic attack), and peripheral vascular disease. A type 2 diabetic is two to four times more likely to suffer myocardial infarction, stroke, and peripheral vascular disease than a nondiabetic. Stroke is responsible for about 15% of all deaths in type 2 sufferers.

Microvascular Complications
Type 1 and 2 diabetes frequently produce similar microvascular complications. Microvascular complications occur probably as a direct result of hyperglycemia and increased blood flow. This causes widespread microvascular damage, and leads to nephropathy, neuropathy, retinopathy, and cardiomyopathy.

Retinopathy
Retinopathy is the most common complication and affects all patients who suffer from diabetes over 20 years. High retinal blood flow, caused by hyperglycemia, induces microangiopathy in capillaries, precapillary arterioles (exposure after 6 years), and venules, causing occlusion and leakage. Retinopathy is a marker for cardiovascular disease, although it is a risk factor for fatal heart attack, only when age and sex were adjusted for.

Nephropathy
Nephropathy, caused by both type 1 and type 2 diabetes, is the result of progressive damage to the small blood vessels. It is signaled by microalbuminuria and later as proteinuria. The resultant impairment of renal function can exacerbate hypertension, thereby establishing a spiral of worsening damage. Two thirds of those with proliferative retinopathy will also have nephropathy. Overt nephropathy takes about 5 to 15 years to develop and affects one

quarter of type 2 diabetic sufferers. The cumulative risk of proteinuria after 20 years of type 2 diabetes is 27%, and the cumulative risk of renal failure after 3 years of proteinuria is over 40%. In type 2 diabetes, albuminuria predicts renal failure and coronary disease. Patients with nephropathy have a greatly increased risk of CVD. Early detection is possible by estimation of the urinary albumin/creatinine ratio. If protein in the urine has been detected and if it is due to diabetes, the average time to onset of renal failure and requirement for dialysis is approximately 8 years, though this varies from patient to patient. Approximately 35% of patients with type 1 diabetes of 18 years' duration will have signs of diabetic renal involvement.[7]

Neuropathy

Diabetes causes mainly peripheral neuropathy, which leads to soft tissue damage and chronic ulceration and finally to gangrene. The severity of neuropathy depends on the duration of diabetes and the degree of its control. It is becoming apparent that autonomic neuropathy makes an important contribution to cardiovascular death. Up to 40% of people with type 1 diabetes who develop abnormalities of autonomic function die within 5 years; 7% of newly diagnosed patients with type 2 diabetes between the ages 25 and 65 have impaired vibration perception in the feet, indicative of neuropathy. Peripheral neuropathy affects half of all type 2 diabetics over the age of 60.

Cardiomyopathy

One reason for the poor prognosis in patients with both diabetes and ischemic heart disease is an enhanced myocardial dysfunction, leading to accelerated heart failure (diabetic cardiomyopathy). Several factors probably underline diabetic cardiomyopathy: severe coronary atherosclerosis, prolonged hypertension, chronic hyperglycemia, microvascular disease, glycosylation of myocardial proteins, and autonomic neuropathy.

Q: How does proteinuria help in stratification of risk and how to manage it?

Macroalbuminuria or proteinuria is defined as urinary albumin excretion of more than 300 mg per liter or per 24 hours (210 µg/min), whereas microalbuminuria refers to urinary albumin excretion between 30 (21 µg/min) and 300 mg per 24 hours. In practice, a macroalbuminuria can be detected as 200 mg/g creatine and microalbuminuria as 30–200 mg/g creatine on spot urine. The important cause of microalbuminuria is diabetes, though it may occur in various disorders such as hypertension and dyslipidemia. Microalbuminuria is present in 30% of middle-aged patients with either type 1 or type 2 diabetes. Among diabetics, it reflects systemic vascular damage and an increased risk of CHD independently of renal function.

Micro- and macroalbuminuria are associated with an increased risk of renal failure, stroke, and cardiovascular mortality.[9] The Monitoring Trends and Determinants of Cardiovascular Disease (MONICA) study established that albuminuria was a potent predictor for the development of ischemic heart disease, independent of other traditional risk factors, such as male gender, hypertension, lipids, advancing age, and obesity.[9] Proteinuria can be regarded as a surrogate marker for atherosclerosis and CVD.

It is suggested that microalbuminuria should be redefined according to the level that increases risk of CHD and CVD[10] as urinary albumin excretion more than 4.8 μg/min (corresponding to 6.4 μg/min during the daytime). Klausen et al. observed that a urinary albumin excretion rate >4.8 μg/min (corresponding to 6.4 μg/min during the daytime) strongly predicts CHD and death, and the predictive effect is independent of age, sex, renal function, diabetes, hypertension, and lipid levels. Data from the HOPE study implied that any degree of microalbuminuria predicts CHD in a patient with or without diabetes.

There is now strong evidence that the renin-angiotensin system is involved in the development of diabetic nephropathy, and that the inhibition of this system slows its progression independently of any antihypertensive effect. A number of meta-analyses have confirmed that angiotensin-converting enzyme (ACE) inhibitors significantly reduce the progression of proteinuria and increase the chance of regression to normoalbuminuria in patients with type 1 diabetes.[11] Two years of ACE inhibitor treatment reduces albumin excretion rates by 50% compared with placebo. The HOPE study showed that in type 2 diabetics with microalbuminuria, ramipril slowed the reduction in the progression to overt nephropathy.[12] In a study of over 4000 patients with type 1 diabetes and proteinuria, treatment with captopril for 3 years led to a 50% reduction in a combined end point of death, dialysis, and transplantation.[13] There is strong evidence that ARBs are renoprotective. They are beneficial for renal outcome and doubling serum creatinine concentration, around a 51% reduction in progression rates from micro- to macroalbuminuria and about a 42% increase in regression from micro- to normoalbuminuria. A study showed that irbesartan can slow or reverse the progression of microalbuminuria to proteinuria, and thus angiotensin receptor blockers (ARBs) can delay the progression of diabetic nephropathy in patients with proteinuria and can reduce all-cause mortality.[15] In a losartan study there was a 16% reduction in the number of patients in the treatment group reaching primary outcome (renal events).[16] Irbesartan and losartan both have been licensed in the U.K. for use in the treatment of renal disease with hypertension and type 2 diabetes.

Q: How does diabetes stratify cardiovascular risk in CHD?

In diabetes, atherosclerosis is accelerated, and there is subsequent resultant cardiovascular morbidity and mortality, often before the age of 50 years. The problem is made worse because the clinical presentation of cardiac disease is altered, making diagnosis more difficult. The risk factors of CHD such as hypertension and dyslipidemia occur more often in diabetics than nondiabetics. Hyperglycemia has been implicated in mechanisms of increased oxidative stress by reversible glycosylation of protein amino groups. The occurrence of the metabolic syndrome in diabetics is well substantiated. In diabetics procoagulant factors play a crucial role. Oxidative stress and endothelial dysfunction in diabetics results in deficient production of prostacyclin and plasminogen activator inhibitor, and is also responsible for increased platelet production of thromboxane A^2.[17] This causes increased vasoconstriction and thrombotic response to plaque rupture and the risk of myocardial infarction (MI). The Framingham study showed that diabetes independently increased the relative risk of CHD by 66% in men and 203% in women followed for 20 years.[18] The risk of acute MI (AMI) in diabetics is 50% higher in men and 150% higher in women. Diabetes also makes it more likely for AMI to occur throughout the day and throughout the year, unlike in a nondiabetic in whom these episodes are likely to occur at specific times, such as in the morning. There is also an increased risk of silent MI (because of the alteration of presenting symptoms), frequency of reinfarction, and restenosis after angioplasty. Also, the complications of AMI are increased in diabetics, particularly heart failure, probably due to more extensive disease rather than the size of the infarct. The cause of diabetic cardiomyopathy, however, is unclear. Sudden death in a diabetic person is more common probably due to increased risk of plaque disruption.

Various studies show that in a diabetic, blood pressure should be controlled more rigidly, ACE inhibitors should be used to reduce cardiovascular risk, and insulin therapy should be used to reduce mortality in diabetic MI. Blood sugar should be more tightly controlled and smoking cessation has greater importance.

Q: Does hyperlipidemia in diabetics needs to be treated differently than in nondiabetics?

It is known from UKPDS that there are several risk factors that are common to CHD and diabetes, such as dyslipidemia (raised LDL-C, low HDL), hypertension, hyperglycemia, and smoking.[2] It is therefore essential that the management of diabetes should also focus on the management of these factors. In both type 1 and type 2 diabetes, the blood level of lipids is similar to those of the general population. As a result, most patients with diabetes do not receive lipid-lowering drugs except those who suffer from dyslipidemia and preexisting CHD. The tendency has been to focus attention on blood sugar and blood pressure control rather than on the lipids. Furthermore, despite the normal or nearly normal levels of LDL-C, the shift to a lipid profile dominated by highly atherogenic small dense LDL-C particles makes people with diabetes suitable for lipid-lowering drugs.[2]

The Greek Atorvastatin and Coronary Heart Disease Evaluation (GREACE) study conducted a trial on 1600 patients with preexisting CHD.[19] One group received the usual care (i.e., advice on lifestyle changes and a lipid-lowering drug as necessary), and the other group was treated with atorvastatin 10 mg daily but titrated (mean dose 23.7 mg daily) to reach a target LDL-C of 2.6 mmol/L (100 mg/dL), which is lower than the current U.K. target of 3 mmol/L. The latter group had a reduced total mortality rate of 43%, CHD mortality was reduced by 47%, and stroke by 47%. Subgroup analysis of the 313 diabetic patients enrolled in this study showed that those in the atorvastatin group had a relative risk reduction of 58%, all-cause mortality reduction of 52%, and stroke reduction of 68%.[20] This trial reemphasized the importance of lowering lipids in diabetics with preexisting CHD.

The Collaborative Atorvastatin Diabetes Study (CARDS) reduced the death rate by 27% (stroke risk by 48% and cardiovascular risk by 37%).[21] No excess of adverse events was noted in the atorvastatin group. Atorvastatin 10 mg daily is safe and efficacious in reducing the risk of first cardiovascular disease event, including stroke, in patients with type 2 diabetes without high LDL cholesterol. No justification is available for having a particular threshold level of LDL cholesterol as the sole arbiter of which patients with type 2 diabetes should receive statins. The debate about whether all people with this disorder warrant statin treatment should now focus on whether any patients are at sufficiently low risk for this treatment to be withheld.

The Veterans Affairs High-Density Lipoprotein Cholesterol Intervention Trial (VA-HIT) study enrolled men with preexisting

CHD and a dyslipidemia similar to that found in diabetes (low HDL and an average LDL).[22] Patients were randomized to the fibrate derivative gemfibrozil or to placebo. After 5 years of treatment, the gemfibrozil group showed a 22% reduction in nonfatal MI or death from cardiac cause. The benefit was similar in patients with diabetes. The Heart Protection Study (HPS) found that statins are successful at reducing cardiovascular events in diabetics and that there is benefit in primary prevention among people with diabetes.[23] Patients treated with simvastatin 40 mg daily showed reduction of a first major cardiovascular event by 25%.

MANAGEMENT

Q: What are the nonpharmacological interventions indicated in the management of diabetes?

The National Institute for Clinical Excellence (NICE) guidelines recommend that patients with type 2 diabetes should have their blood pressure and blood lipids checked annually. Lifestyle measures need to be adhered to. The role of increased physical activity, weight reduction, and smoking cessation cannot be overemphasized.

Regular exercise reduces the risk of developing type 2 diabetes. The greater the frequency of activity, the higher the protection from diabetes. To achieve this aim, the exercise program has to last for more than a year, and probably up to 4 years.[24]

High blood pressure and raised lipids needs to be treated by lifestyle modification or therapeutic agents. Microalbuminuria and lipids should be tested annually and glycated hemoglobin biannually (target <7%). It is more important to treat these conditions in hypertensive patients as they further increase the risk of CVD. The American Diabetic Association (AHA) recommends low-dose aspirin as a secondary prevention strategy and a primary prevention strategy in those who have high risk of CVD. Clopidogrel has been demonstrated to reduce CVD rates in diabetes. Adjunct therapy in very high risk patients or as an alternative to aspirin in intolerant patients should be considered.

Dietary Measures

A diabetic diet is not any different from a healthy diet. The organization Diabetes UK recommends that the meal plate should contain the following food items[25]:

- Half the plate should contain vegetables, salads, and fruits.
- One sixth of the plate should contain meat, fish, and beans.
- Two sixths of the plate should contain rice, pasta, and potatoes.

Sugar intake does not have to be stopped completely. Consumption of fat and total carbohydrates is more important. Sucrose can provide up to 10% of daily energy requirements, provided it is taken as part of a healthy diet. Sugar in food does not give rise to any more additional problems with blood sugar control, because sugar does not raise blood sugar levels any more than the same amount of calories in the form of starch. However, sugary drinks, such as some fruit squash and fruit drinks, and certain foods rich in sugar, such as chocolate and cakes, should be avoided. It is advisable that the person consumes low-sugar versions of foods. Sweeteners such as saccharine (e.g., Sweetex), aspartame (e.g., Canderal, Nutrasweet), acesulfame K (e.g., Sweet-n-Low 2), cyclamate, and sucralose can be used instead of sugar.

Not much emphasis has been laid on fiber intake in the recent recommendations from Diabetes UK. Soluble fiber has beneficial effects on blood sugar and lipid control. Insoluble fiber has no direct effect on blood sugar and lipid metabolism but is useful for weight reduction. Monosaturated fats should form the main source of dietary fats because they are less harmful in the development of atheroma.

Glycemic Index

A diabetic should eat carbohydrates with a low glycemic index (GI). The GI is a ranking of carbohydrate-containing foods based on their overall effects on blood sugar levels. Slowly absorbed foods have a low GI rating, and foods that are more quickly absorbed have a higher GI rating. Many factors influence the GI, such as cooking method, processing, the ripeness of fruit, and the variety of vegetable. The addition of fat and protein also affects the GI. Fats and proteins slow the absorption of carbohydrates by increasing the gastric emptying time. It is recommended that a combination of high- and low-GI food should be eaten. For instance, combining a jacket potato (high GI) with baked beans (low GI) gives a medium-GI meal.

Diabetes UK recommends that a person should choose carbohydrate foods with a low GI more often as part of a meal, for example, beans, peas and pulses, spaghetti, barley, low-fat milk and milk products, and starchy foods such as pasta, basmati rice, noodles, sweet potatoes, plantain, and pita bread. (Table 3.3). The total quantity of dietary carbohydrates has the biggest impact on blood sugar levels. The GI was originally produced to help diabetics reduce postprandial peaks of glucose but was shown to be positively associated with CHD in the Nurses' Health Study.

TABLE 3.3. Glycemic index (GI) of some common foods

Food	GI
Kellogg's All Bran	51
Kellogg's Corn Flakes	84
Oatmeal	49
Basmati rice	58
Brown rice	55
Noodles (instant)	46
Spaghetti	43
Bagel	72
Doughnut	76
Milk (whole)	22
Yogurt (low fat)	33
Apple	38
Banana	55
Grapefruit	25
Orange	44
Broccoli	10
Mushroom	10
French fries	73
Potato (baked)	93
Lentils	30
Glucose	100
Pretzels	83

Q: How do oral hypoglycemic drugs differ in their mode of action and indications?

There are five types of oral hypoglycemic agents (Table 3.4):

1. Biguanides (i.e., metformin)
2. Thiazolidinediones (insulin sensitizers)
3. Sulfonylureas
4. α-Glycosidase inhibitors (i.e., acarbose, miglitol)
5. Meglitinides (prandial glucose regulators)

Physicians should prescribe drugs that target insulin resistance, such as metformin and thiazolidinediones. Both these drugs lower triglycerides, but pioglitazone has the advantage that it also raises HDL-C without significantly increasing LDL-C.

Biguanides

Biguanides exert their effect mainly by decreasing gluconeogenesis and by increasing peripheral utilization of glucose. They also

TABLE 3.4. Oral hypoglycemic agents

Generic	Daily dose (maximum single dose)	Fre	Comments
Sulfonylureas			
Glibenclamide	2.5–15 mg (15 mg)	1	*Side-effects*: hypoglycemia, weight gain, hepatic
Chlorpropamide*	250–750 mg (750 mg)	1	toxicity, blood dyscrasias. *Contraindications*: severe
Gliclazide	40–80 mg (160 mg)	1–2	hepatic/renal disease, porphyria, with insulin,
Glimepiride	1–4 mg (6 mg)	1	pregnancy, lactation
Glipizide	2.5–20 mg (15 mg)	1–3	
Gliquidone	45–60 mg (60 mg)	2–3	
Glyburide*	1.2–20 mg	s/d	
Biguanides			
Metformin	500–3000 mg (1 g)	1–3	*Side-effects*: GI upset, lactic acidosis. *Contraindications*: hepatic & renal disease, pregnancy, lactation
Meglitinides			
Nateglinide	60–180 mg (180 mg)	1–3	*Side-effects*: keto-acidosis. *Contraindications*:
Repaglinide	0.5–16 mg (4 mg)	1–3	pregnancy & lactation. To be taken before each meal
Thiazolidinediones			
Pioglitazone	15–30 mg (45 mg)	1	Monitor for heart and liver problems
Rosiglitazone	4–8 mg (8 mg)	1	
α-Glucosidase inhibitors			
Acarbose	50–600 mg (200 mg)	1–3	*Side-effects*: flatulence
Miglitol	25–100 mg (100 mg)	3	

* Not in U.K.; s/d, single or divided; Fre, frequency.

impair glucose absorption in the gut. Metformin, the only bigu-anide available in the U.K., should be the initial monotherapy for all overweight people, and should be considered as an option for initial monotherapy even in those who are not overweight (BMI <25 kg/m^2). Metformin targets the whole cardiovascular risk, and patients treated with metformin had a lower risk of MI compared to patients treated with intensive therapy with insulin.[30] Metformin can be used in combination with other oral agents and insulin. Diarrhea can result from taking too high a dose of metformin too quickly or not taking this drug with or after food. Renal function tests (serum creatinine, urea, and electrolytes) should be done before initiating therapy and then should be repeated annually.

Metformin can be taken when there is impaired glucose toler-ance, gestational diabetes, obesity accompanied with high blood pressure, and raised lipids. In the Diabetic Prevention Program (1984–2001), metformin therapy prevented or delayed the onset of type 2 diabetes in persons with impaired glucose tolerance. If insulin therapy is started, metformin should be continued, and orli-stat may be considered as part of the weight reduction program.

Thiazolidinediones (Pioglitazone and Rosiglitazone)
Thiazolidinediones improve insulin-mediated glucose disposal by enhancing sensitivity to insulin in the liver, adipose tissue, and skeletal muscle. They increase insulin-stimulated uptake and storage of glucose and reduce breakdown of triglycerides to produce free fatty acids. This reduces glucose output from the liver and causes muscles to use glucose preferentially, further lowering blood levels. They have a favorable effect on blood pressure, dys-lipidemia, and possibly on CHD outcome. Either drug can be used for initiating monotherapy in overweight patients. Pioglitazone can lower cholesterol by 15%.[26] Pioglitazone and rosiglitazone can be used with sulfonylurea or metformin, but the combination with metformin should be preferred. If a patient fails to respond to com-bination therapy of metformin and sulfonylurea, then insulin should be used.

Sulfonylureas
Sulfonylureas act mainly by increasing insulin secretion from the pancreas, but may also act at extrapancreatic sites to enhance the activity of insulin. Therefore, they are effective only when some beta cells are still present. Sulfonylureas are no longer the drug of choice in type 2 diabetes. Gliclazide is the most suited sulfomylu-rea especially in the elderly as there is less risk of renal failure. Chlorpropamide (no longer recommended) and glibenclamide are

usually avoided in the elderly due to the risk of hypoglycemia. Tolbutamide and glipizide cause fewer hypoglycemic events than chlorpropamide and glibenclamide. Glipizide can be used in addition to metformin, if the latter is unable to control blood sugar alone. When the combined cotherapy with strict diet and sulfonylurea fails, sulfonylureas can be used in combination with metformin, acarbose, and thiazolidinediones or with bedtime isophane insulin.

α-Glucosidase Inhibitors: Acarbose

Complex carbohydrates, which form part of dietary carbohydrates, have to be broken down into monosaccharides by a group of enzymes called α-glucosidases before their absorption in the gut. Acarbose inhibits the action of α-glucosidase, thereby reducing the release of monosaccharides into the bloodstream, thus preventing postprandial hyperglycemia. It can be used alone or in conjunction with sulfonylureas and biguanides.

Prandial Glucose Regulators, Meglitinides

Nateglinide and repaglinide are nonsulfonylurea oral hypoglycemic agents that stimulate the release of insulin from the pancreas. They are taken just before each main meal. As they have a rapid onset and a short duration of action, insulin is secreted when blood glucose levels are at their highest but not when they are low. Thus, they reduce blood sugar spikes after meals and are less likely to cause hypoglycemia. Repaglinide can be used alone or as an add-on/alternative to metformin in non-obese patients. Nateglinide is licenced in USA only with metformin.

Hemoglobin A_{1c} should be measured every 2 to 6 months when diabetes is unstable and then every 6 months thereafter. The target level of HbA_{1c} should be 6.5% to 7.5% based on microvascular and macrovascular complications. When glycemic control is unsatisfactory, another agent should be added and not substituted.

Q: Can the onset of diabetes be delayed?

There is now substantial evidence that type 2 diabetes can be prevented or delayed. It is not yet known whether the successful intervention can cost-effectively reduce the mortality and morbidity associated with diabetes. Insulin resistance develops 20 to 30 years before the onset of diabetes. Targeting insulin resistance can therefore postpone the onset of diabetes. In the management of insulin resistance, the risk factors should be targeted, such as hypertension, diabetes, obesity, dyslipidemia, and smoking. Insulin resistance can be reduced within a few days of introducing a low-calorie diet even before much weight loss has occurred.[7] Subsequent weight loss further improves insulin sensitivity. Exercise, especially vigorous exercise, reduces insulin resistance, although this effect is lost quickly (within 5 days) if exercise stops.[7,27] In the treatment of hypertension, beta-blockers and thiazides should be avoided, as they exacerbate insulin resistance, whereas ACE inhibitors and α-blockers reduce it. The cardioprotective and renoprotective action of ACE inhibitors or ARBs is independent of blood pressure reduction. These protective effects are achieved through various mechanisms, such as their effects on the endothelium and the arterial wall. Aspirin should be prescribed unless contraindicated. Metformin and thiazolidinediones should be preferred over other oral antidiabetic agents, as they reduce insulin resistance.

Metformin has been shown to reduce risk of developing type 2 diabetes in individuals with impaired glucose tolerance, but prescribing it has not become standard practice.

The biguanide metformin reduced the risk of diabetes by 31% in the Diabetes Prevention Program,[29] and acarbose reduced the risk by 32% in the study to prevent non–insulin-dependent diabetes mellitus (STOP-NIDDM) trial.

Q: Is sildenafil safe to use in a diabetic man who has erectile dysfunction?

Erectile dysfunction is a common problem in diabetic men. It affects 55% of 60-year-old men with diabetes. Sildenafil citrate, a selective inhibitor of cyclic guanosine monophosphate (cGMP)-specific phosphodiesterase type 5, is the first new class of oral agents effective in the treatment of erectile dysfunction of various causes. Normal penile erection is mediated by the nitric oxide (NO)–cGMP pathway. In response to sexual stimulation, neurons and arteriolar endothelial cells of the corpus cavernosum of the penis release NO. This neurotransmitter stimulates the formation of cGMP, which in turn leads to the relaxation of vascular and trabecular smooth muscle and dilatation of penile blood vessels. Since sildenafil and nitrates both cause cGMP-induced vasodilatation, their concurrent use can lead to a significant fall in blood pressure.

Sildenafil can be taken in the initial dose of 50 mg (25 mg in the elderly) approximately 1 hour before sexual activity. Subsequent doses are adjusted, according to the response, from 25 to 100 mg as a single dose (maximum 100 mg in 24 hours). Sildenafil is well tolerated and its side effects are mild. This group of drugs should be used with caution in patients with cardiovascular disease or anatomical deformation of penis (e.g., Peyronie's disease, angulation, cavernosal fibrosis). Sildenafil is contraindicated with nitrates, recent myocardial infarction, and if blood pressure is less than 90/50 mm Hg. Although sildenafil is a gold standard, its effect may be slowed for about 2 hours if taken after a meal, especially when alcohol has been consumed. Normally, on an empty stomach, sildenafil works after 35–40 minutes. Other newer drugs of similar action are tadalafil, vardenafil, and Levitra. The absorption of tadalafil and Levitra is not affected by food and alcohol. Tadalafil can be given in the dose of initially 10 mg, approximately 30 minutes to 12 hours before sexual activity, with subsequent doses adjusted, according to the response, up to 20 mg. The action lasts for 24 hours. Contraindications and side effects of these drugs are similar to those of sildenafil.

References

1. WHO database, 2003. www.who.int.
2. Turner RC, Millins H, Neil HA, et al. Risk factors for coronary artery disease in non-insulin dependent diabetes mellitus. United Kingdom Prospective Diabetes Study (UKPDS: 23). BMJ 1998;316:823–828.
3. Multiple Risk Factor Intervention Trial. Risk factor changes and mortality results. JAMA 1982;248:1465–1477.
4. Grundy S, Becker D, Clarke L, et al. National Cholesterol Education Program (Adult Treatment Panel 111). Detection, education, and treatment of high blood cholesterol in adults. Circulation 2002;106: 3143–3420.
5. Wallace AM, McMohan AD, Pickard CJ, et al. Plasma leptin and the risk of cardiovascular disease in West of Scotland Coronary Prevention Study. Circulation 2001;104:3052–3056.
6. Ridker PM, Wilson WF, Grundy SM. Should CRP be added to metabolic syndrome and to the assessment of global cardiovascular risk? Circulation 2004;109:2818–2825.
7. Grundy SM, Benjamin IJ, Burke GL, et al. Diabetes and cardiovascular disease. Circulation 1999;100:1134–1146.
8. Borch Borch-Johnsen K, Feldt-Rasmussen B, Strandgaard S, et al. Urinary albumen excretion: an independent predictor of ischemic heart disease. Arterioscler Throm Vasc Biol 1999;19:1992–1997.
9. Cohn JM, Quyyumi AA, Hollenberg NK, et al. Surrogate markers for CVD. Circulation 2004;109(suppl):1V-37-46.
10. Klausen, Borch-Johnsen K, Feldt-Rasusson B, et al. Very low levels of microalbuminuria are associated with increased risk of CHD and death independently of renal function, hypertension and diabetes.
11. Kshirsagar AV, Joy MS, Hogan SL, et al. Effects of ACE inhibitors in diabetic and non-diabetic chronic renal disease: a systematic overview of randomized placebo-controlled trials. Am J Kidney Dis 2000;35: 695–707.
12. Heart Outcome Prevention Evaluation (HOPE) Study Investigators. Effects of ramipril on cardiovascular and microvascular outcomes in

people with diabetes mellitus: result of HOPE study and MICRO-HOPE substudy. Lancet 2000;355:253–259.

13. Lewis EJ, Hunsicker LG, Bain RP, et al. The effects of angiotensin-converting-enzyme inhibition on diabetic nephropathy. The Collaborative Study Group. N Engl J Med 1993;329:1456–1462.

14. UK Prospective Diabetes Study (UKPDS) Group. Effect of intensive blood-glucose control with metformin on complications in overweight patients with type 2 diabetes (UKPDS 34). Lancet. 1998;352(9131): 854–865.

15. Lewis EJ, Hunsicker LG, Clarke WR, et al. Renoprotective effects of the angiotensin-receptor antagonist irbesartan in patients with nephropathy due to type 2 diabetes. N Engl J Med 2001;345:851–860.

16. Brenner BM, Cooper ME, de Zeeuw D, et al. Effects of losartan on renal and cardiovascular outcome in patients with type 2 diabetes and nephropathy (RENNAL study). N Engl J Med 2001;345:861–869.

17. Davi G, Ciabottoni G, Consoli A, et al. In vivo formation of 8-iso-prostaglandin F2a and platelet activation in diabetes mellitus: effects of improved metabolic control. Circulation 1999;99:224–229.

18. Kannel WB, McGee DL. Diabetes and cardiovascular risk factors: the Framingham Study. Circulation 1979;59:8–13.

19. Athyros VG, Papageorgiou AA, Mercouris BR, et al. Treatment with atorvastatin to the National Educational Program goal vs "usual care" in secondary CHD prevention. The Greek Atorvastatin and Coronary Heart Disease Evaluation (GREACE) Study. Curr Med Res Opin 2002; 18;220–228.

20. Athyros VG, Papageorgious AA, Symeonidis AN, et al. Early benefit from structured care with atorvastatin in patients with coronary heart disease. Angiology 2003;54:679–960.

21. Thomason MJ, Colhoun HM, Livingstone SJ, et al, the CARDS Investigators. Baseline characteristics in the Collaborative AtoRvastatin Diabetes Study (CARDS) in patients with type 2 diabetes. Lancet 2004; 21:685–696.

22. Rubins HB, Robins SJ, Collins D, et al. Gemfibrazil for the secondary prevention of coronary heart disease in men with low levels of high-density lipoprotein cholesterol. Veterans Affairs High-Density Lipoprotein Cholesterol Intervention Trial Study Group. N Engl J Med 1999; 341:410-418.

23. Collins R, Armitage J, Parish S, et al. MRC/BHF Heart Protection Study of cholesterol-lowering with simvastatin in 20, 536 high risk individuals:a randomised placebo-controlled trial. Lancet 2002;360:7–12.

24. Obesity in Scotland. Integrating prevention with weight management. A National Clinical Guideline Guideline 55. Scottish Intercollegiate Guidelines Network (SIGN) Edinburgh, 2000.

25. Diabetes UK. www.diabetes.org.uk.

26. Khan ME, St. Peter JV, Xue J. Prospective randomized comparison trial of the metabolic effects of pioglitazone or rosiglitazone in patients with type 2 diabetes who were previously treated with troglitazone. Diabetes Care 2002;25:708–711.

27. American Diabetes Association. Consensus Development Conference on Insulin Resistance. Diabetes Care 1998;21:310–314

28. Buchanan TA, Xiang AH, Peters RK, et al. Preservation of pancreatic B-cell function and prevention of type 2 diabetes by pharmaceutical treatment of insulin resistance in high risk Hispanic women. Diabetes 2002;51:2796–2803.

29. Chiasson JL, Gomis R, Hanefield M, et al. The STOP-NIDDM trial. Acarbose for the prevention of type 2 diabetes. Lancet 2002; 359:2072–2077.

30. Knower WC, Barrett-Conner E, Flower SE, et al. Diabetic Prevention Program. Reduction in the incidence of type 2 diabetes with lifestyle intervention or metformin. N Engl J Med 2002;346:393–403.

Chapter 4

Hypertension

Hypertension is defined as systolic blood pressure (BP) ≥140 mm Hg or diastolic BP ≥90 mm Hg or when the individual is taking an antihypertensive agent. There is a direct relationship between hypertension and coronary heart disease (CHD), and new evidence reinforces the importance of high blood pressure as a risk factor for cardiovascular disease (CVD) in men and women. The incidence of CHD among individuals with hypertension is equal to all other adverse outcomes combined. Severe hypertension may directly damage arterioles and cause atherosclerosis. High blood pressure is also a risk factor for stroke. The risk of cardiovascular events is increased two to three times in men and women with hypertension. It is estimated that 14% of deaths from CHD in men and 12% of deaths from CHD in women are due to hypertension. In people over the age of 50 years, systolic BP of >140 mm Hg is a more important CVD risk factor than diastolic BP. Beginning at BP 115/75 mm Hg, the CVD risk doubles for each increment of BP of 20/10 mm Hg; those who are normotensive at 55 years of age have a 90% lifetime risk of developing hypertension.[1,2]

DIAGNOSIS AND ASSESSMENT

Q: What is abnormal blood pressure and up to what age it should be checked?
The British Hypertension Society's (BHS) classification of blood pressure levels has changed in line with recent European guidelines (Table 4.1). Hypertension up to the age of 80 years should be treated. It is unclear if there is any advantage in doing so above the age of 85 years. However, ongoing studies should make it clear in the future. In the meantime, all adults should have their blood pressure measured every 3 years until the age of 80 years. People with high normal systolic (130–139 mm Hg) or diastolic blood pressure (85–89 mm Hg) and people who have had a high blood pressure reading at anytime previously should have their blood pressure measured annually.

TABLE 4.1. Classification of hypertension (British Hypertension society and U.S. Joint National Committee [JNC7])

Category	BP (mm Hg)			
	Systolic		Diastolic	US equivalent category
Optimal	<120	and	<80	Normal
Normal	<130	and	<85	Prehypertension*
High-normal	130–139	or	85–89	Prehypertension*
Hypertension				
Grade 1 (mild)	140–159	or	90–99	Stage I**
Grade 2 (moderate)	160–179	or	100–109	Stage II†
Grade 3 (severe)	≥180	or	≥110	Stage III†

JNC 7 recommendations without compelling indications:
* Drugs for compelling indication.
** Thiazide-type diuretics for most; may consider ACE inhibitor, ARB, beta-blocker, CCB, or combination.
† Two-drug combination for most (usually thiazide-type diuretic and ACE inhibitor or ARB or beta-blocker or CCB).

Q: What is nocturnal hypertension and what are the indications of ambulatory blood pressure monitoring (ABPM) in clinical practice?
There is a normal fluctuation of blood pressure during the day, and at night when the blood pressure dips. Even among most hypertensives, the BP dips (by at least 20%), but even those in whom such a dip is not present (nocturnal hypertension nondippers) are at increased risk of cardiovascular events. Of all hypertensives, 5% are nondippers, and of these 40% have secondary hypertension. Twenty-four-hour blood pressure recording will differentiate dippers from nondippers.

The "white-coat" effect (white-coat hypertension) is a condition in which blood pressure is raised in the presence of a doctor or nurse but falls when the person leaves the office. Ambulatory blood pressure monitoring correlates better than office measurements with target organ damage. Young adults who show a large BP response to psychological stress may be at risk of hypertension as they approach midlife.[3]

The BHS guidelines for ambulatory blood pressure monitoring are as follows:

• Unusual variability of blood pressure.
• Possible white-coat hypertension.
• Informing equivocal treatment decisions.

- Evaluation of nocturnal hypertension (nondippers).
- Evaluation of drug-resistant hypertension.
- Determining the efficacy of drug treatment over 24 hours.
- Diagnosis and treatment of hypertension during pregnancy.
- Evaluation of symptomatic hypertension.

Q: Is systolic, diastolic, or pulse pressure a better prognostic indicator? Should isolated hypertension be treated?

Both systolic and diastolic readings of blood pressure are important, but systolic BP is a better predictor of events (CHD, CVD, heart failure, stroke, end-stage renal disease, all-cause mortality), especially in an older person. Risk of cardiovascular accident is more closely related to systolic hypertension (raised systolic reading >160 mm Hg), while diastolic BP is more important until 50 years of age. In fact, the pulse pressure (the difference between systolic and diastolic blood pressure), particularly in elderly women, may be a strong predictor of cardiovascular events, in addition to absolute systolic and diastolic blood pressure measurements. A pulse pressure of more than 70 indicates increased cardiovascular risk.

Isolated systolic hypertension (ISH) is defined as a systolic blood pressure >160 mm Hg in association with a normal diastolic blood pressure of less than 90 mm Hg. In the Systolic Hypertension in Elderly People (SHEP) trial, after an average of 4.5 years treatment, a reduction in mean systolic blood pressure of only 11 mm Hg resulted in 36% fewer strokes and 27% fewer fatal and nonfatal heart attacks in the elderly treated group.[4] The benefit was also evident across all ages, all races, both sexes, and all BP subgroups.

Q: What is the target blood pressure and at what level should high blood pressure be treated? Is there any truth in the J-shaped curve theory?

The BHS recommends that the target systolic BP for most patients should be ≤140 mm Hg and the diastolic ≤85 mm Hg, whereas for patients with diabetes, renal disease, or established CVD, it should be SBP ≤130 mm Hg and diastolic ≤80 mm Hg.[5] The BHS also recommends the use of drug therapy in patients with sustained grade 2 hypertension (i.e., systolic ≥160 mm Hg or sustained diastolic ≥100 mm Hg). All patients with grade 1 hypertension (systolic BP 140–159 or diastolic BP 90–99, or both) should also be offered antihypertensive drugs, if there is any hypertensive complication, target organ damage, or diabetes, or if there is an estimated 10-year risk of CVD of ≥20%, despite lifestyle changes. In diabetics, drug treatment should be initiated if the sustained systolic BP is

≥140 mm Hg or the sustained diastolic BP is ≥90 mm Hg. The "audit standard" for clinical purposes in the U.K. is systolic BP <150 mm Hg and diastolic <90 mm Hg for a nondiabetic, and systolic BP <140 mm Hg and diastolic <80 mm Hg for a diabetic patient. The recommendations of the American Diabetic Association are described elsewhere in Chapter 3. Target organ damage includes:

- Left ventricular hypertrophy, myocardial infarction (MI), angina, revascularization, and heart failure.
- Stroke or transient ischemic attack (TIA).
- Peripheral vascular disease.
- Retinopathy.
- Renal impairment (raised serum creatinine), proteinuria.

J-Shaped Curve Theory

The J-shaped curve theory that it is dangerous to reduce blood pressure too low is no longer accepted, and this is supported by the Hypertension Optimal Treatment (HOT) study.[6] Now, trials with aggressive blood pressure lowering drugs show safety and huge benefits. The diastolic blood pressure should not be lowered to <55 mm Hg but in practice this is rarely a problem. The HOT study suggests that the optimal blood pressure for reduction of major cardiovascular events was 139/83 mm Hg and that reduction of blood pressure below this level causes no harm, but no further reduction of cardiovascular (CV) events is achieved. In diabetics, however, reducing diastolic BP to 81 mm Hg decreased CV events. Recent research, however, suggests the lower the better.

Q: What is the benefit of reducing blood pressure?

Trials show that an average treatment produces fall in diastolic blood pressure of 5 to 6 mm Hg, which was associated with a highly significant reduction in fatal and nonfatal stroke (38%) and fatal and nonfatal heart attack (16%); there was, however, no difference in individual trials. Lowering of normal blood pressure also does not confer any benefit. The absolute reduction depends on the initial level of cardiovascular risk. The benefits of blood pressure reduction could be summarized as follows:

- Prevent stroke (approximately 40%) and MI (approximately 20%).
- Reduce target organ damage.
- Decrease progression of heart failure (especially in the elderly) or atrial fibrillation.
- Improve prothrombotic states.

MANAGEMENT

Q: What steps should be taken when high blood pressure is diagnosed?
If hypertension is suspected or diagnosed, the following steps should be taken:

- Assess cardiovascular risk factors and complications.
- Determine the identifiable causes of hypertension.
- Assess the presence of target organ damage.
- Conduct a history and physical examination.
- Investigate the findings.
- Offer advice on lifestyle modification interventions.
- Offer advice on primary or secondary prevention.
- Initiate drug therapy, if indicated.

Risk Factors for Cardiovascular Disease
Major risk factors: smoking, hypertension, raised low-density lipoprotein (LDL)-C, diabetes, low high-density lipoprotein (HDL) (independently predicts the risk of CVD), age.
Underlying factors: obesity/overweight, physical inactivity, atherogenic diet, socioeconomic and psychological stress, family history, and various genetic factors.
Emerging factors: various lipid factors (triglycerides, apolipoproteins, lipoprotein [a], lipoprotein subfractions). Nonlipid factors include insulin resistance, prothrombotic markers, and proinflammatory markers.

Secondary Causes of Hypertension
- Pregnancy: blood pressure may rise in the latter part of pregnancy, preeclampsia.
- Kidney diseases: renal artery stenosis, polycystic kidneys, chronic pylonephritis, glomerulonephritis, polyarteritis nodosa, systemic sclerosis, systemic lupus erythematosis, immunoglobulin A (IgA) nephropathy, obstructive uropathy.
- Endocrinal diseases: pheochromocytoma, Cushing's syndrome, hypothyroidism, thyrotoxicosis, hyperparathyroidism, Conn's syndrome (primary aldosteronism), acromegaly, and congenital adrenal abnormalities.
- Drug-related/induced: corticosteroids, estrogen-containing drugs (e.g., contraceptive pill), nonsteroidal antiinflammatory drugs, and sympathomimetics.
- Food induced: liquorice.
- Miscellaneous: coarctation of aorta, sleep apnea.

Resistance hypertension may be due to improper BP measurement, inadequate anthypertensive dose, poor compliance, excessive salt or alcohol intake, drug interaction, white-coat hypertension, or secondary to an underlying cause.

History and Physical Examination

The history and physical examination can often give clues to the underlying cause, and it also helps to plan the investigations and subsequent management of patients. Pointers for secondary hypertension include clinical symptoms and signs, such as palpable kidneys (polycystic kidneys, adrenal tumor), delayed or absent femoral pulses (aortic coarctation), truncal obesity or pigmented striae (Cushing' syndrome), hypokalemia (hyperaldosteronism), hematuria and proteinuria (nondiabetic renal disease), paroxysmal tachycardia, sweating (pheochromocytoma), resistance hypertension, and abnormal results of routine tests.

Investigations (Table 4.2)

Life Modification Measures

Lifestyle-modifying recommendations should be enforced. The Dietary Approaches to Stop Hypertension (DASH) trial showed that a diet that emphasizes fruits, vegetables, and low-fat dairy products; that includes whole grains, poultry, fish, and nuts; and that contains only a small amount of total and saturated fat and cholesterol, lowers blood pressure substantially both in hyperten-

TABLE 4.2. Investigations in hypertension

First-line investigations
   Urine: for protein, sugar, and blood
   Blood: for urea, electrolytes, creatinine, lipids, liver function test,
      thyroid function test
   Electrocardiogram

Further investigations
   Echocardiography assesses left ventricular hypertrophy/dysfunction
   24-hour ambulatory BP if diagnosis in doubt
   Estimated glomerular filtration rate for chronic renal disease
   24-hour urinary metanephrine and normetanephrine for
      pheochromocytoma
   24-hour urinary aldosterone level for primary aldosteronism
   Doppler flow study, resonance angiography for renovascular
      hypertension
   Parathyroid hormone for parathyroid disease
   Sleep study with oxygen saturation for sleep apnea

sives and nonhypertensives, as compared to a typical U.S. diet.[7] The second DASH trial, in which sodium intake was lowered and intake of K, Ca, and Mg was increased, found a combined effect of Na reduction and the DASH diet that was greater than a single effect.[8] When the DASH diet is combined with low sodium (2.4 or 1.8 g), greater reduction of blood pressure is achieved. In overweight patients, there is approximately a 1 mm Hg fall in blood pressure for each 1 kg of weight loss. Reducing salt intake from 12 to 6 g daily results in a reduction of the systolic/diastolic blood pressure by about 5/2–3 mm Hg. Regular exercise such as brisk walking for 30 minutes for most days reduces systolic blood pressure by 4 to 9 mm Hg. Healthy diet reduces systolic BP by 2 to 8 mm Hg, and limiting alcohol intake to no more than two drinks a day will drop the systolic BP by 2 to 4 mm Hg.[1,9] Similarly, other measures such as smoking cessation cannot be ignored. Primary and secondary prevention is described in Chapter 6.

Pharmacological Options

There are six groups of drugs that are recommended as first- or second-line agents for the treatment of high blood pressure. Most patients need two or more antihypertensive agents. In fact, in the HOT study, it took up to five drugs to achieve control.[6] In many cases, lower doses of two or more agents are better tolerated. The drugs need to be chosen carefully, taking into account of the patient's age, ethnicity, race, and cultural beliefs, and the presence of other risk factors. The following groups of drugs are used for the treatment of hypertension:

1. Diuretics, e.g., thiazide (bendrofluazide).
2. Beta-blockers, e.g., atenolol.
3. Calcium channel blockers, e.g., amlodipine, felopidine, etc.
4. Angiotensin-converting enzyme (ACE) inhibitors, e.g., lisinopril, ramipril.
5. Angiotensin-11 blockers, e.g., losartan.
6. Alpha-blockers, e.g., doxazosin (others are prazosin, indoramin, terazosin).

Q: What is the role of diuretics in hypertension and what is the evidence?

Thiazide diuretics and related drugs, such as chlortalidone, inhibit sodium reabsorption at the beginning of the distal convoluted tubule of kidney. Recent guidelines recommend that low-dose thiazides (e.g., bendrofluazide 2.5 mg) should be used as a first-line drug in hypertension unless there is a compelling reason not to do so or there is reason to use another drug. The antihypertensive effect of thiazides is not dose dependent. They are especially effective in elderly patients, including those with systolic hypertension. Thiazides also reduce all-cause mortality. Low-dose thiazide diuretic therapy has also been endorsed by the seventh report of the Joint National Committee (JNC)[1] as the first-line monotherapy in hypertensive older persons. The huge Antihypertensive and Lipid-Lowering Treatment to Prevent Heart Attack Trial (ALLHAT) study showed that thiazide diuretics are a vital and important class of drug for treating high blood pressure and remain as first-line agents for many years.[10] Side effects of thiazides include disturbance of blood sugar, cholesterol, or uric acid, and impotence. Other thiazides (clopamide, cyclopenthiazide, hydrochlorothiazide, hydroflumethiazide) do not offer any significant advantage over bendrofluazide and chlortalidone. Chlortalidone (chlorthalidone) and hydrochlorothiazide are prescribed in the dose of 25 to 50 mg daily in the morning and can be combined with a potassium-sparing diuretic.

Indapamine is related to chlorthalidone and is prescribed in the dose of 1.5 to 2.5 mg daily. It is indicated for the treatment of mild to moderate hypertension and has less metabolic disturbance, particularly less aggravation of blood sugar and uric acid. Spironolactone, although not licensed for the management of hypertension in the U.K., is now recommended by the BHS in step four of its guidance. It is used in the dosage of 25 mg daily. Furosemide (Frusemide) is not regarded as antihypertensive but can potentiate ACE inhibitors. It can be used as an alternative to thiazides, if renal function is impaired (serum creatinine >160 μmol/L).

ALLHAT Study
This study showed that thiazide (chlorthalidone), lisinopril, and amlodipine were equally good at preventing fatal or nonfatal cardiac events. It also suggested that alpha-blockers might be inadvisable as a first-line therapy. The doxazosin limb of the ALLHAT study was discontinued due to an increasing trend toward congestive heart failure compared to the chlorthalidone group. In practice alpha-blockers are most used when calcium-channel blockers or ACE inhibitors are unsuccessful or inappropriate.

Q: How do beta-adrenoceptor blocking drugs differ in their actions and what are their indications?
Beta-adrenoceptors of the sympathetic nervous system are of two types: beta-1 and beta-2. The division of beta-blockers into cardioselective (blocking largely beta-1 receptors in the heart) and

noncardioselective (blocking both beta-receptors) is relative; even the most cardioselective beta-blocker has some blocking effect on the beta-2 receptor. Cardioselective agents at low dosage are relatively beta-1 specific. Beta-1 blockade slows the heart rate, reduces myocardial contractility, and reduces cardiac output and the cardiac workload. It thus reduces myocardial demand, and improves coronary perfusion, hence relieving cardiac ischemic pain. Blockage of beta-2 receptors causes vasodilatation and bronchospasm. Beta-blockers also reduce renin in the blood (which reduces angiotensin); therefore, they work well with diuretics and vasodilators. They control arrhythmias by directly acting on the heart. Beta-blockers are used in the treatment of angina, hypertension, arrhythmias, thyrotoxicosis, anxiety, migraine, and post-myocardial infarction (Table 4.3).

First-generation beta-blockers (oxprenolol, propranolol) are noncardioselective and generally well tolerated, although they may produce peripheral ischemia, central nervous system (CNS) disturbance, or bronchospasm, or exacerbate congestive heart failure and reduce exercise tolerance. They also adversely affect plasma lipids and reduce hepatic glucose mobility. Second-generation

TABLE 4.3. Beta-blockers

Generic name	Daily dosage	Side effects and contraindications
Cardioselective		*Side effects*: Cold extremities,
Atenolol	50–100 mg	exacerbation of PVD, lethargy,
Metoprolol m/r	200 mg	sleep disturbance, nightmares, depression, impotence, heart
Acebutolol	200 mg bid	weight gain, bronchospasm,
Celiprolol	200–400 mg	failure, rash, exacerbation of
Bisoprolol	5–20 mg	psoriasis, lipid and glucose
Betaxolol	10–40 mg	disturbance; contraindications:
Noncardioselective		bronchial asthma or history of
Propranolol	80–160 mg bid	bronchospasm, uncontrolled
Nadolol	80–240 mg	heart failure, Prinzmetal's
Nebivolol	2.5–5 mg	angina, marked bradycardia, low blood pressure, heart
Timolol	5–20 mg bid	block, severe PVD, and
Carvedilol	12.5–25 mg	pheochromocytoma,
Penbutolol	20 mg	co-prescribing with diltiazem
Oxprenolol m/r	160 mg	or verapamil
Pindolol	5–30 mg	
Labetatol	50–400 mg bid	

m/r = modified release.

beta-blockers (e.g., atenolol, bisoprololol, metoprolol) have greater cardioselectivity and a lesser, but still somewhat adverse effect on triglycerides and HDL cholesterol. The third-generation beta-blockers (e.g., celiprolol, nebivolol) have a peripheral vasodilating effect and do not affect lipid levels adversely. As with more selective drugs, those with intrinsic sympathomimetic activity (e.g., acebutol, oxprenolol, pindolol) are less likely to cause cold extremities and produce less effect on resting heart rate and cardiac output.

Q: Are calcium channel blockers safe and effective as compared to other antihypertensive?

Calcium channel blockers (CCBs, calcium antagonists) interfere with the inward calcium displacement of calcium ions through the slow channels of active cell membrane. They cause peripheral and coronary vasodilatation, and reduce myocardial contractility. There are three categories of CCBs (Table 4.4): phenylalkylamine, dihydropyridine, and benzothiazepine. Verapamil and diltiazem are chemically distinct from each other and also from all the other calcium-channel blockers that come under the category of dihydropyridines. Verapamil and diltiazem share many properties with beta-blockers, such as blocking electrical impulses through the conducting system. Verapamil slows atrioventricular node conduction and reduces myocardial contractibility, and hence is useful as an antiarrhythmic drug. Verapamil and diltiazem are contraindicated in heart failure and in those patients taking beta-blockers or digoxin. In fact, most CCBs exacerbate symptoms of heart failure. Amlodipine may be a safer option in these patients. Dihydropyridines (amlodipine, etc.) do not resemble beta-blockers, but are potent vasodilators and can be safely co-prescribed. The older short-acting CCBs such as nifedipine may cause rapid dilatation, reflex tachycardia, and catecholamine surges, and may worsen myocardial ischemia. Therefore, slow-release preparations of nifedipine or a long-acting formulation such as amlodipine should be used.

In the elderly, hypertensive CCBs reduce mortality. These are the drugs of choice for patients with asthma or peripheral vascular disease (PVD). The CCBs have no adverse effect on lipids, glucose, or sexual function. They reverse left ventricular hypertrophy (LVH) and are particularly effective where there is renal damage and in African Caribbeans (whose renin level is low).

A study showed CCBs and ACE inhibitors to be equally effective in regressing LVH.[11] Although ACE inhibitors are the drugs of choice in hypertension with diabetes, CCBs are suitable as add-on agents for many patients who require two or more drugs to control

TABLE 4.4. Calcium channel blockers

Generic name	BP	Angina	Daily dose	Fre	Comments
Dihydropyridines					
Amlodipine	√	√	2.5–10 mg	1	*Side-effects*: headache, flushing, ankle swelling. *Contraindication*: short-acting nifedipine not to use in angina & hypertension. *Caution*: sudden withdrawal may exacerbate angina
Felopidine	√	√	2.5–10 mg	1	
Nicardipine sust/re	√	√	60–120 mg	2	
Nifedipine long acting	√	√	30–60 mg	1	
Nisoldipine	√	√	10–40 mg	1	
Isradipine	√	x	1.25–5 mg **	2	
Lacidipine	√	x	2–6 mg	1	
Lercanidipine	√	x	10–20 mg	1	
Nondihydropyridines					
Phenylalkylamine-verapamil immediate release	√	√	240–360 mg	3	Verapamil: also used in arrhythmias, may impair AV conduction, avoid in heart failure. *Contraindicated* with beta-blocker: Avoid diltiazem with beta-blocker and in heart failure. *Side-effects*: bradycardia. Withdraw slowly
verapamil long acting	√	√	120–480 mg	1–2	
Benzothiazepine-diltiazem	√	√	180–360 mg	3	
diltiazem extended release	√	√	120–420 mg	1	

**B also CR 1 daily; Fre, frequency; x, not indicated; √, indicated.

blood pressure. The Fosinopril Versus Amlodipine Cardiovascular Events Randomized Trial (FACET) showed that treatment with fosinopril reduced the risk of CV events more effectively than amlodipine, but that the combination of an ACE inhibitor and a CCB was more effective in reducing the risk of CV events than either agent alone.[12] Amlodipine is effective as the ACE inhibitor (cilazapril) in lowering progression of renal disease over 3 years in patients with type 2 diabetes and hypertension, whether or not there is evidence of nephropathy when treatment was initiated.[13]

The Systolic Hypertension in Europe study found that treatment with CCBs eliminated the excess risk of CV disease associated with diabetes.[14] This finding is consistent with those of the HOT randomized trial, which found that the benefits of treatment with CCBs, with or without an ACE inhibitor or a beta-blocker, and with the possible addition of a diuretic, were greater among patients with diabetes. In these patients, the group whose target blood pressure was 80 mm Hg or less had the risk of major CV events reduced by half, CV mortality by two thirds, and total mortality by 43%, compared to the group whose target blood pressure was 90 mm Hg or less.

Q: What is the mechanism of action of ACE inhibitors and what are their advantages over other drugs?

Renin-Angiotensin-Aldosterone System

The renin-angiotensin-aldosterone system is one of the mechanisms that maintains normal blood pressure (Fig. 4.1). Renin is an enzyme produced by cells in the kidneys, and it releases angiotensin I from renin substrate (angiotensinogen) produced in the liver. Angiotensin-converting enzyme (ACE) converts angiotensin I into a potent form called angiotensin II. It also converts bradykinin, substance P, and the tachykinins into inactive fragments. However, angiotensin is also formed in the tissues via non-ACE pathways, in which both angiotensinogen and angiotensin I are converted directly to angiotensin II by enzyme other than ACE.

The ACE inhibitors prevent the conversion of angiotensin I to angiotensin II. They also block the destruction of bradykinin, the accumulation of which causes cough and angioedema. They cause reduction of blood pressure through a reduction in peripheral vascular resistance and, to a lesser extent, through prevention of the renal absorption of sodium by aldosterone. They may also improve endothelial function and reduce central adrenergic tone. Their potency broadly compares to that of diuretics and beta-blockers. They achieve sustained blood pressure reductions of 11/10 mm Hg

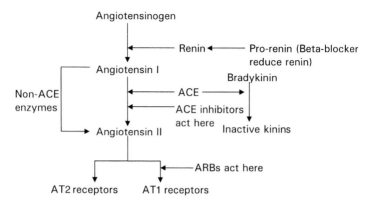

FIGURE 4.1. The renin-angiotensin system and site of action of angiotensin-coverting enzyme (ACE) inhibitors and angiotensin receptor blockers (ARBs).

(systolic/diastolic) over 4 years. ACE inhibitors are effective hypertensives in 40% to 50% of patients when used as monotherapy. When ACE inhibitors are first started, patients need to be supervised carefully. There is a useful synergism among the ACE inhibitors, diuretics, and CCBs. Renal function tests should be done before starting the drug and repeated a few weeks after. If there is a rise in serum creatinine, the drug should be stopped. ACE inhibitors reverse left ventricular hypertrophy more than other antihypertensives. It is now firmly established that ACE inhibitors are superior to other drugs used in the treatment of hypertension in reducing micro- and macroalbuminuria, and progression of renal disease in diabetic patients. ACE inhibitors are also beneficial in nondiabetic patients with proteinuria and kidney damage. They have no adverse effects on lipids or blood glucose level. On the contrary, there is some evidence that they have a beneficial effect on insulin resistance. ACE inhibitors are also the drugs of choice in patients with heart failure, whether or not associated with hypertension (Table 4.5).

If a patient is already receiving diuretic therapy, the ACE inhibitors should be started at a low dosage (due to hypovolemia), and diuretic therapy may have to be discontinued for 24 hours beforehand. ACE inhibitors may cause a rapid fall in blood pressure, particularly in those receiving diuretic therapy; the first dose should preferably be given at bedtime. Potassium-sparing diuretics should be discontinued before starting ACE inhibitors because of the risk

TABLE 4.5. Angiotensin-converting enzyme (ACE) inhibitors

BP	Heart failure	Post-MI	Generic name	Daily dose mg	Frequency (daily)	Comments
✓	✓	✓	Enalapril	2.5–40	1	*Side effects*: dry cough, renal impairment, angioedema, rash, rhinitis, GI upset, altered liver function, blood disorders, first-dose hypotension; *caution*: risk of hyperkalemia with potassium-sparing diuretics, risk of profound hypotension to a patient on loop diuretic, temporary withdrawal of loop diuretic reduces the risk; renal function monitored; not to use in pregnancy renovascular disease, or with NSAIDs
✓	✓	✓	Lisinopril	10–40	1	
✓	✓	✗	Perindopril	4–8	1	
✓	✓	✗	Quinapril	20–80	1	
✓	✓	✓	Ramipril	2.5–10	1	
✓	✓	✗	Fosinopril	10–40	1	
✓	✓	✗	Cilazapril	1.5	1	
✓	✓	✓	Trandolapril	1–4	1	
✓	✗	✗	Moexipril	7.5–30	1	
✓	✓	✓	Captopril	25–100	2	
✓	✗	✗	Benazepril	10–40	1	

of hyperkalemia. Reducing salt intake can have a beneficial effect with ACE therapy. The Heart Outcome Prevention Evaluation (HOPE) study showed that ramipril reduces the rate of death, MI, stroke, revascularization, cardiac arrest, heart failure, complications related to diabetes, and new cases of diabetes in a broad spectrum of high-risk patients.[15] Only a small part of the benefit was attributed to the hypotensive effect, as the reduction in blood pressure was extremely small (2–3 mm Hg). Among African Caribbeans, hypertension occurs despite low levels of renin (low-renin hypertension). Therefore, this type of hypertension does not respond to drugs that affect the renin angiotensin cycle.

Q: How do angiotensin II receptor blockers differ from ACE inhibitors in their mode of action, efficacy, and benefits?

Angiotensin II, an octapeptide derived from its inactive precursor angiotensin I by the action of ACE, is the final product of the renin-angiotensin system. Angiotensin II is a significant contributor to the pathogenesis of arterial disease, hypertension, left ventricular hypertrophy, heart failure, and renal disease. It exerts its effects by stimulating cell membrane receptors, which are subtyped into ATI and AT2 receptors. Almost all recognized affects of angiotensin II are mediated by the AT1, receptors, which are blocked by ATI receptor antagonist drugs. Stimulation of AT1 receptor causes severe vasoconstriction and enhanced sympathetic nervous system activity, and increases the release of aldosterone and antidiuretic hormone. This increases blood pressure, retains sodium and water, and adversely affects cardiovascular function and structure. The function of the AT2 receptor is poorly defined, but it is thought to be involved in the growth and differentiation during embryonic development. Angiotensin receptor blockers (ARBs) act on the renin-angiotensin-aldosterone system, where they block the action of angiotensin II at its receptors.

The ARBs do not block AT2 receptors and may in fact cause their stimulation because plasma angiotensin is raised. However, stimulation of AT2 receptors in the presence of an AT1 receptor blockage may produce benefit rather than harm, because AT2 receptors appear to mediate antiproliferative effects and may even attenuate the proliferative effects of AT1 receptor stimulation. This suggests that ARBs may be better than ACE inhibitors. In addition, unlike ACE inhibitors, ARBs do not interfere with bradykinin, substance P, or tachykinin metabolism, thus avoiding class-specific side effects of the ACE inhibitors. This is because the ACE enzyme has a greater affinity for bradykinin than it does for angiotensin I. The disadvantage may be that bradykinin is likely to mediate the

TABLE 4.6. Angiotensin II receptor blockers

Generic name	Frequency (daily)	Daily doses	Comments
Losartan	1–2	25–100 mg	Use with *caution* in renal
Valsartan	1–2	80–320 mg	artery stenosis, elderly,
Irbesartan	1	150–300 mg	renal impairment; monitor
Candesartan	1	8–32 mg	plasma K;
Eprosartan	1–2	400–800 mg	*contraindications* as
Telmisartan	1	20–80 mg	withACE inhibitors
Olmesartan	1	20–40 mg	

adverse effects of cough and perhaps angioedema and cate-cholamine release. The advantage may be that bradykinin is likely to stimulate nitric oxide and prostacyclin release, which should improve endothelial function and may even be antiatherosclerotic. AT2 receptor stimulation, however, might have harmful effects.[2]

Since angiotensin II is a trophic substance, it is more likely to prevent or regress left ventricular hypertrophy as compared to other antihypertensives. Olmesartan (20 mg) has been compared to candesartan (8 mg) and found to reduce daytime and 24-hour diastolic and systolic blood pressure more effectively than candesartan at the doses tested[16] (Table 4.6).

Additive effects have been reported when used with thiazides and with beta-blockers. The onset of action is gradual, and only rarely is there risk of first-dose hypotension. The ARBs are well tolerated, including by elderly patients, but caution needs to be exercised when the patient is already on diuretics. They are suitable for patients who develop a cough with ACE inhibitors, but may become first-line drugs in their own right in due course. The plasma concentration of potassium tends to rise slightly, and therefore the concomitant use of potassium supplements or potassium-sparing diuretics is not advocated. There is also the potential for an adverse interaction with nonsteroidal antiinflammatory drugs, precipitating renal failure.

The antihypertensive effect of losartan is not dose dependant, unlike other ARBs. However, all ARBs provide 24-hour blood pressure control. Serum potassium and creatinine should be tested before commencing angiotensin II antagonists, and 4 weeks after. In patients with hypertension and type 2 diabetes mellitus or renal damage, ARBs are associated with preservation of renal function and reduction of microalbuminuria (Chapter 3). Indications, contraindications, and side effects are similar to those for ACE inhibitors, except that AT2 blockers do not cause cough, angioedema, and altered taste. However, sporadic cases of angio-edema have been reported.

The ARBs are recommended by the American Diabetic Association as the first-line treatment for diabetics with diabetic nephropathy following the results from trials such as the Irbesartan Patients with Type 2 Diabetes and Microalbuminuria (IRMA-2),[17] Microalbuminuria Reduction with Valsartan (MARVAL),[18] Irbesartan Diabetic Nephropathy Trial (IDNT),[19] and Reduction of Endpoints in non–insulin-dependent diabetes mellitus (NIDDM) with the Angiotensin II Antagonist Losartan (RENNAL).[20] These studies show that ARBs have renal benefits beyond and possibly unrelated to the lowering of BP. A study showed that telmisartan 40 or 80 mg once daily was well tolerated in the treatment of mild to moderate hypertension, producing sustained 24-hour blood pressure control, which compared favorably with losartan.[21]

LIFE Study
The Losartan Intervention for Endpoint reduction (LIFE) study randomized over 9000 hypertensive patients with left ventricular hypertrophy (1195 with diabetes) to losartan or atenolol.[22] ARBs were found to have substantially better outcome than atenolol in patients with left ventricular hypertrophy for nearly identical blood pressure lowering. The difference in cardiovascular events in the losartan group was largely attributable to a risk reduction in stroke despite there being little difference in BP between the groups. This raises the possibility of stroke prevention with ARBs.

SCOPE Trial
Candesartan has also been shown in the study on cognition and prognosis in the elderly (SCOPE) trial to have an important benefit over existing conventional antihypertensive therapy in the reduction of risk of stroke in elderly hypertensives, especially if they have left ventricular hypertrophy or diabetes.[23]

ACE Inhibitors and ARBs Combination
In the candesartan and lisinopril microalbuminuria study, the combination of an ACE inhibitor and ARBs produced a greater blood pressure reduction and lower albumin urinary excretion loss than either treatment alone, in patients with hypertension, diabetes, and microalbuminuria.[24]

Q: What is the present strategy for selecting antihypertensive agents, when used alone or in combination?
The British Heart Society (BHS) provides guidelines on combinations using an A (ACE inhibitor or ARBs), B (beta-blockers), C

(calcium channel blockers), or D (diuretics) system.[25] Younger patients respond better to A or B drugs, whereas older patients or African Carribeans respond better to C or D drugs. When combining drugs, it is logical to use a second agent from the other groups (i.e. A + C or B + D, etc.) (Fig. 4.2). A beta-blocker with an ACE inhibitor or ARB is not an ideal combination due to a similar mechanism of action on the renin-angiotensin system. Similarly, a CCB with a thiazide diuretic is not good due to a similar action of vasodilatation. The following recommendations are based on the seventh JNC report.[1]

When There Is No Compelling Indication
Where BP is more than 20 mm Hg above the systolic goal or more than 10 mm Hg above the diastolic goal, the Adult Treatment Panel (ATP) 111 recommends initiating treatment with two drugs, one of which should be a thiazide or related drug. For stage 1 hypertension, prescribe a thiazide for most patients, and consider ACE inhibitors, ARBs, beta-blockers, or CCBs alone or in combination. For stage 2 hypertension, initiate a combination of two drugs, usually a thiazide and an ACE inhibitor or ARBs, or a beta-blocker or CCB.

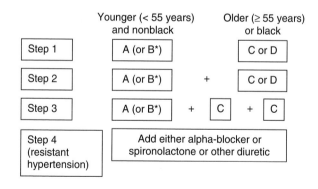

A: ACE inhibitor or angiotensin-II antagonist
B: beta-blocker
C: calcium channel blocker
D: diuretic (thiazide)
*Combinations of B and D may induce more new-onset diabetes compared with other drug combinations.

FIGURE 4.2. British Hypertension Society (BHS) recommendations for combining antihypertensive drugs. "British Medical Journal, BMJ 2004:328: 637–640, amended and reproduced with permission from the BMJ Publishing Group."

When There Are Compelling Indications for Individual Drug Classes

- Post-MI: beta-blocker, ACE inhibitor, and aldosterone antagonist.
- Angina and silent MI: beta-blocker; if contraindicated a CCB should be added or substituted.
- Ischemic heart disease: beta-blocker first, alternatively CCB.
- Acute coronary syndrome: initially beta-blocker and ACE inhibitor.
- High cardiovascular disease risk: thiazide diuretic, beta-blocker, ACE inhibitor, and CCB are beneficial.
- Diabetes: thiazide type, beta-blocker, ACE inhibitor, ARB, and CCB are useful in reducing CVD and stroke in diabetic hypertensive. ACE inhibitors and ARBs delay renal function deterioration.
- Heart failure: for asymptomatic with ventricular dysfunction, use ACE inhibitor and beta-blocker. For symptomatic ventricular dysfunction or end-stage heart failure, use ACE inhibitor, beta-blocker, ARB, and aldosterone antagonist with loop diuretic.
- Chronic kidney disease: if the glomerular filtration rate (GFR) <60 mL/min, then ACE inhibitor and ARB. In more advanced renal disease (GFR <30 mL/min), increase the dose of the loop diuretic in combination with other drugs.
- Cerebrovascular disease: recurrent strokes are reduced by ACE inhibitors and thiazides.
- Blacks: reduced response to monotherapy with beta-blockers, ACE inhibitors, or ARBs compared with diuretics and CCBs. Drug combination can reduce this problem.
- Pregnancy: methyldopa, beta-blockers (i.e. labetalol), and vasodilators are safer.

Q: What are the criteria of treating hypertension in diabetes?
Hypertension, a known CHD risk factor for diabetics, is present in 30% to 50% of patients with type 1 diabetes and up to 70% of patients with type 2. Even a slight rise of blood pressure in a diabetic, which may be within normal limits for a nondiabetic, may be serious due to incipient diabetic nephropathy. There appears to be risk of hypertension in both type 1 and type 2. In type 1 diabetes, hypertension may be present at onset, later become normalized, and then return during the first 5 to 10 years after the onset of diabetes. However, in type 2 diabetes, hypertension is part of a wider problem of insulin resistance. Diabetic children, however, have a higher systolic blood pressure from adolescence onward. Patients with diabetes derive more absolute benefits from blood pressure reduction than do nondiabetics.

Type 1 Diabetes

Hypertension in a patient with type 1 diabetes is a good predictor of diabetic nephropathy and macrovascular disease. Type 1 diabetics, in the absence of incipient nephropathy (absence of microalbuminuria) have a similar incidence of hypertension as nondiabetics. However, the incidence of hypertension increases in the presence of microalbuminuria; therefore, it can be stated that all type 1 diabetics with hypertension have underlying nephropathy. Incipient nephropathy leads to frank nephropathy, and eventually to renal failure. To prevent renal damage, tighter control of blood pressure is essential, and to accomplish that, more than two hypertensive agents may be required.

Type 2 Diabetes

Hypertension is very common in type 2 diabetes and is present in 40% of cases at initial diagnosis. The presence of high blood pressure in type 2 diabetics does not always indicate renal involvement; this is in contrast to type 1 diabetics. Obesity may be a major factor linking hypertension with diabetes, which may be the case because both diabetes and hypertension have similar predisposing genetic and environmental factors. There is some evidence of a higher incidence of hypertension among relatives of type 2 diabetics, indicating the familial-essential nature of the disease. The high blood pressure may be detected even before the onset of diabetes, which may be precipitated by thiazide later.

UKPDS Study

The United Kingdom Prospective Diabetic Study (UKPDS)[26] and the Hypertension Optimal Treatment (HOT) trial[5] emphasized the importance of tighter control of blood pressure. The UKPDS randomized over 5000 patients in 23 centers, with a mean blood pressure of 160/94 with type 2 diabetes. One group was treated intensively and the other less so. After 20 years of study, it was noted that the group that was intensively treated for blood pressure showed a reduced incidence of all macrovascular (nonfatal and fatal) complications by 34%, stroke by 44%, and heart attack by 21%. Moreover, there was a 37% reduction in diabetic microvascular complications. Diabetes-related deaths were reduced by 32%, but there was no significant reduction in all-cause mortality. A high proportion of patients with diabetes require three or more agents (a third at 8 years in the UKPDS) to achieve adequate control.

The choice of the drug in the treatment of hypertension in type 2 diabetes is an ACE inhibitor or beta-blocker, though the UKPDS did not find any significant difference in the outcome by using different drugs, which included ACE inhibitors, beta-blockers, low-dose thiazides, and dihydropyridines (e.g., amlodipine).

Treatment of Hypertension in Diabetes

The American Diabetes Association recommendations include the following[27]:

- Diastolic blood pressure should be lowered to <80 mm Hg. If the diastolic blood pressure is 80 to 89 mm Hg, lifestyle/behavioral therapy should be advised initially for 3 months; if the target is not achieved, drug therapy should be started. If the diastolic blood pressure is ≥90 mm Hg, the patient should receive drug therapy in addition to lifestyle/behavioral therapy.
- If the systolic blood pressure is 130 to 139 mm Hg, lifestyle/behavioral therapies should be advised initially for 3 months; if the target (130 mm Hg) is not achieved, drug therapy should be started. If the systolic blood pressure is ≥140 mm Hg, the treatment should be initiated with drug therapy in addition to lifestyle/behavioral therapy.
- ACE inhibitors, beta-blockers, and diuretics should be used initially in uncomplicated hypertension, as these have been shown to reduce cardiovascular events.
- If the patient has type 1 diabetes, with or without hypertension, with any degree of albuminuria, ACE inhibitors have been shown to delay the progression of nephropathy.
- In patients with type 2 diabetes, hypertension, and microalbuminuria, ACE inhibitors and ARBs have been shown to delay the progression to macroalbuminuria.
- In patients with type 2 diabetes, hypertension, macroalbuminuria, nephropathy, or renal insufficiency, ARBs should be strongly considered, unless contraindicated.
- In patients over 55 years of age with or without hypertension but with another risk factor (dyslipidemia, microalbuminuria, smoking, history of CVD), an ACE inhibitor should be considered to reduce the risk of CVD.

Q: What is the importance of 24-hour blood pressure control?

It is important that blood pressure is controlled throughout the day. The peaks of death from coronary artery disease and cerebrovascular accidents (e.g., stroke, TIA), and incidents of sudden death seem to occur between the hours of 6 a.m. and midday. It is, therefore, essential that the antihypertensive effect of the drugs should last until the effect of the next dose comes into force so as to give protection during the early hours of morning. The complications of hypertension are likely if blood pressure is not controlled over the 24-hour period. Most patients have their blood pressure measured in the morning after they have taken their morning dose of antihypertensive drug. It is possible that blood pressure is controlled with the peak effect of the drug at that time but providing inadequate protection toward the end of the day or the next morning.

The so-called trough/peak ratio is put forward as a guide by the U.S. Food and Drug Administration as a means to determine what percentage of a drug's effectiveness persists over the 24-hour period. This ratio is affected by many factors such as the dose of drug and the rate at which it is metabolized. It appears that when a drug has a trough/peak ratio of greater than 70%, only then is it likely to give 24-hour control of blood pressure. Of the ACE inhibitors, perindopril, trandolapril, and ramipril can be taken once a day, but enalapril, and captopril need to be taken more than once a day to control BP for 24 hours. Thiazides, atenolol, most ARBs, and amlodipine can be taken once a day.

References

1. Chobanian A, Bakris GL, Black H, et al. Seventh report on the Joint National Committee on Prevention, Detection, Evaluation, and Treatment of High Blood Pressure. Hypertension 2003;42:1206–1252.
2. Levy B. Can angiotensin II type 2 receptors have deleterious effects in cardiovascular disease. Circulation 2004;109:8–13.
3. Mathews KA, Katholi R, McCreath H, et al. Blood pressure reactivity to psychological stress predicts hypertension in the CARDIA study. Circulation 2004;110:74–78.
4. SHEP Cooperative Research Group. Prevention of stroke by antihypertensive drug treatment in older person in isolated systolic hypertension. Final result of the Systolic Hypertension in Elderly Program (SHEP). JAMA 1991;265:3255–3264.
5. Williams B, Poulter NR, Brown MJ, et al. British Hypertensive Society guidelines for hypertension management 2004 (BSH-1V): summary. BMJ 2004;328:634–640.
6. Hansson L, Zanchetti A, Carruthers SG, et al., for the HOT Study Group. Effects of intensive blood-pressure lowering and low-dose aspirin in patients with hypertension: principal results of the Hypertension Optimal Treatment (HOT) randomized trial. Lancet 1998;351: 1755–1762.
7. Apple LJ, Moore JJ, Oberzanek E, et al. DASH Collaborative Research Group. A clinical trial of the effects of dietary pattern on blood pressure. N Engl J Med 1997;336:1117–1124.
8. Kesteloot H. Epidemeological studies on the relationship between, Na, K, Ca and Mg and arterial blood pressure. J Cardiovasc Pharmacol 1994; 6:S192–S196.

9. Sacks FM, Sverkey LP, Vollmer WM, et al. Effects on blood pressure of reduced dietary sodium and the Dietary Approaches to Stop Hypertension (DASH) diet. N Engl J Med 2001;344:3–10.

10. Furberg CD, Wright JT, Davies BR, et al., on behalf of the ALLHAT Collaborative Research Group. Major outcomes in high-risk hypertensive patients randomized to angiotensive-converting enzyme inhibitor or calcium channel blockers vs diuretic. The Antihypertensive and Lipid-Lowering Treatment to Prevent Heart Attack Trial (ALLHAT). JAMA 2002;288:2981–2997.

11. Schmieder RE, Schlaich MP, Klingbeil A, et al. Reversal of left ventricular hypertrophy in essential hypertension: a meta-analysis of randomised double blind studies. Nephrol Dial Transplant 1998;13:564–569.

12. Tatti P, Pahor M, Byington RP, et al. Outcome results of the Fosinopril vs Amlodipine Cardiovascular Events Randomised Trial in patients with hypertension and non-insulin dependent diabetes mellitus. Diabetic Care 1998;21:597–602.

13. Velussi M, Brocco E, Frigato F, et al. Effects of cilazapril and amlodipine on kidney function in hypertensive NIDDM patients. Diabetes 1996; 45:216–222.

14. Staessen JA, et al. Morbidity and mortality in the Syst-Eur Trial. Lancet 1997;350:757–764.

15. Heart Outcome Prevention Evaluation Study (HOPE). Effects of an angiotensin converting enzyme inhibitor, ramipril, on cardiovascular events in high-risk patients. N Engl J Med 2000;324:145–153.

16. Brunner H. Clinical efficacy of olmesartan medoxmil. J Hypertens 2003;21(suppl 2):s43–s46.

17. Parving H, Lehnhert H, Bröchner-Mortensen J, et al. The effects of irbesartan on the development of diabetic nephropathy in patients with type 2 diabetes. N Engl J Med 2001;345:870–878.

18. Viberti G, Wheeldon NM. Microalbuminuria reduction with valsartan in patients with type 2 diabetes mellitus. A blood pressure-independent effect. Circulation 2002;106:672–678.

19. Lewis EJ, Hunsicker LG, Clarke WR, et al. Renoprotective effects of the angiotensin-receptor antagonist irbesartan in patients with nephropathy due to type 2 diabetes. N Engl J Med 2001;345:851–860.

20. Brenner BM, Cooper ME, de Seeuw D, et al. Effects of losartan on renal and cardiovascular outcomes in patients with type 2 diabetes and nephropathy. N Engl J Med 2001;345:861–869.

21. Mallion BJ, Siche JP, Lacourciere Y, et al. ABPM comparison of anti-hypertension profile of the selected ARBs, telmesartan and losartan in patients with mild to moderate hypertension. J Hum Hypertens 1999; 13:657–664.

22. Dahlof B, Devereux RB, Kjeldsen J, et al. Cardiovascular morbidity and mortality in the Losartan Interventtion for Endpoint reduction in hypertensive study (LIFE): a randomisized trial against atenolol. Lancet 2002;359:995–1003.

23. Hansson L, Lithell H, Skoog I, et al., for SCOPE Trial. Prague: European Society of Hypertension, Blood Press 2000;9:146–151.

24. Mogensen CE, Neldam S, Tikkanen I, et al. Randomised controlled trial of dual blockage of renin-angiotensin system in patients with hypertension, microalbuminuria and non-insulin dependent diabetes: the candesartan and lisinopril microalbuminuria (CALM) study. BMJ 2000;321:1440–1444.

25. Brown MJ, Cruickshank JK, Dominiczak AF, et al. Better blood pressure control: how to combine drugs. J Hum Hypertens 2003;17:81–86.

26. United Kingdom Prospective Diabetic Study Group. Tight blood pressure control and risk of macrovascular and microvascular complications in type 2 diabetes. UKPDS 38. BMJ 1998;317:703–713.

27. Arauz-Pacheo C, Parrot MA, Raskin P, American Diabetes Association. The treatment of hypertension in adult people with diabetes. Diabetes Care 2002;25:134–147.

Chapter 5
Cardiac Investigations

The aim of cardiac investigations in coronary heart disease (CHD) is not only diagnostic but also therapeutic and prognostic. Routine screening of asymptomic patients is not worthwhile. Initial investigations in primary care should include a resting electrocardiogram (ECG), plain chest x-ray, and blood testing for hemoglobin, erythrocyte sedimentation rate (ESR), renal function test, glucose, lipid profile, liver function, and thyroid function test. The cardiac investigation can be invasive or noninvasive. Although with the present noninvasive techniques substantial information regarding both anatomical and physiological information can be gained, it is necessary in some cases to do invasive procedures.

Clinicians have to decide which way to proceed if one test is positive and another negative. Performing additional tests is also of limited value because of predictive redundancy, meaning that the incremental information from performing a second noninvasive test is less than would be expected if the tests were independently predictive.[1] If a patient had a negative test with one modality, there is the likelihood of having the same result with another modality. Similarly, false-positive results with one test are likely to have the same result with another procedure. If a noninvasive test is selected carefully in one patient and the result is borderline, which does not fit with the clinical picture, then performing another noninvasive test may not be helpful. However, all noninvasive tests have considerable prognostic value. New serum markers, including C-reactive protein (CRP) and homocysteine have the ability to gauge risk in the individual patient.

ELECTROCARDIOGRAPHY

Q: What are the indications for 24 hour ambulatory ECG?
Dynamic electrocardiography, also called Holter monitoring or 24-hour ambulatory ECG, is a continuous tape recording of one or more electrocardiographic leads obtained by means of a small

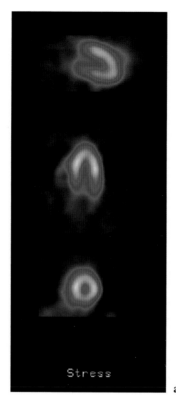

Stress

FIGURE 5.1. A thallium scan. (a) Normal thallium. (b) Thallium-reversible ischemia in left anterior descending (LAD) territory. Reproduced by permission of Dr Arvind Vasudeva, Consultant Cardiologist, Kingston Hospital, Surrey, U.K.

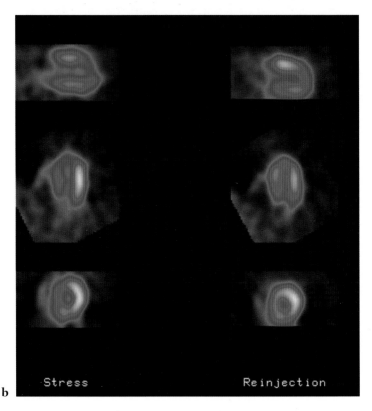

Stress   Reinjection

FIGURE 5.1. *Continued*

portable tape recorder, which remains attached to the patient for 24 hours. The recording is helpful for detecting paroxysmal arrhythmias. The role of ambulatory monitoring has now expanded to assessing antidysrhythmic therapy, detecting myocardial ischemia and assessing prognosis.[2] Chest pain, palpitations, and fainting attacks are some of the other indications.

Q: What are the indications for exercise stress testing in clinical practice, and what are its limitations?

Exercise stress testing (EST), such as the treadmill test and exercise ECG, is done widely for diagnosing angina, which provides both diagnostic and prognostic information, with an average sensitivity of 68% and specificity of 77% in a patient who has cardiac symptoms or hypertension. Testing is usually done on a treadmill but can also be done on a stationary bicycle. American Heart Association (AHA) guidelines advise that a trained physician be present when the test is carried out.[3]

The exercise test is reliable in a population with a high prevalence of coronary artery disease, although when the prevalence is low (e.g., in young women with atypical symptoms) the frequency of false-positive results becomes unacceptably high. The appearance of ventricular tachyarrhythmia or a significant fall in systolic blood pressure during exercise also identifies patients at high risk of a future heart attack, irrespective of ECG changes. The interpretation of EST should include symptomatic response, exercise capability, hemodynamic response and ECG response. The occurrence of ischemic chest pain during testing is highly suggestive of angina, especially if it forces termination of the test.

The Bruce protocol test (variable speed grade exercise test) is based on the work done by R.A. Bruce and is the most popular. It is designed so that the exercise ends within 6 to 15 minutes, an interval that allows patients to warm up and is not too long to cause tiredness. The most commonly used definition of a positive exercise test are when typical anginal discomfort is reproduced, or ≥1 mm of horizontal or down-sloping ST-segment depression, or elevation of ≥60 to 80 ms after the end of the QRS complex. The test is markedly positive if ischemic changes develop in the first 3 minutes of exercise or persist 5 minutes after exercise, if ST depression is ≥3 mm, if systolic BP falls ≥10 mm Hg, or if high-grade ventricular arrhythmia develops. If the patient is able to manage exercise tolerance for more than 9 minutes, it indicates a good long-term prognosis, whereas less than 3 minutes indicates a poor prognosis.[3] The test is terminated when an ST segment shift of more than 0.2 mV (=2 mm) occurs, in the event of chest pain, breathlessness, or fatigue, or on achieving a heart rate of 85% to 90% of the maximum predicted for the patient's age and sex. The test is also discontinued if the systolic blood pressure falls >10 mm Hg or sustained ventricular arrhythmia or ST elevation (≥1 mm) in leads without diagnostic Q-waves (other than V1 or aVR)[3] occurs during exercise. EST, however, is an insensitive predictor of restenosis with sensitivities ranging from 40% to 55%, significantly less than those from single photon emission computed tomography (SPECT).

Treadmill testing when used alone cannot be regarded as an effective screening test for ischemic heart disease. Well-obstructed coronary arteries if accompanied with good collateral circulation may yield a negative exercise test; on the other hand, the treadmill stress test (EST) will produce a high proportion of false-positive tests.

Treadmill testing is poor at reflecting disease in the circumflex territory. Interpretation of the exercise ECG is also difficult if there is a resting bundle branch block or other abnormalities. Indications for stress testing are as follows:

- Confirmation of angina
- Assessment of myocardial ischemia and prognosis
- Assessment of risk stratification after myocardial infarction (MI)
- Evaluation of revascularization procedures

Contraindications of stress testing are as follows:

- Outflow obstruction (e.g., obstructive cardiomyopathies)
- Cardiac failure
- Aortic stenosis or mitral stenosis
- Uncontrolled hypertension
- Recent MI (within 2 days)
- Complete heart block
- Severe arrhythmias
- Systolic hypertension >200 mm Hg and diastolic >100 mm Hg

STRESS ECHOCARDIOGRAPHY

Q: What are the indications for stress echocardiography, and how does it figure in risk stratification?
Drug-induced stress echocardiography is gaining recognition in the United Kingdom as a very useful noninvasive technique to investigate ischemic heart disease. It involves imaging by two-dimensional echocardiography. The Doppler shift effect during ultrasound can

be combined to provide information on the velocity and direction of blood flow. Stress echocardiography also provides assessment of left ventricular function, valvular function, and myocardial ischemia and chamber size. Examination of the heart by stress echocardiography involves producing stress either by exercise or by giving drugs that increase myocardial contraction and heart rate (e.g., dobutamine or arbutamine) or by dilating coronary arteries (e.g., by dipyridamol or adenosine). Dobutamine has emerged as the best alternative to exercise as it is safe and well tolerated and serious side effects are rare. Stress echocardiography is indicated for the assessment of myocardial ischemia and myocardial viability, and for evaluating prognosis. The test relies on the principle that progressive stress will induce myocardial ischemia and reduce contractile function in the area of the affected myocardium. Two-dimensional echocardiogram is recorded at baseline and at stress. Motion abnormalities are recorded in different segments of the left ventricle. Stress echocardiography has a higher sensitivity and specificity than exercise treadmill testing and is useful in patients whose physical condition limits exercise. Stress echocardiography can also be used for detecting myocardial viability, and to differentiate areas of infarcted tissue from hibernating myocardium when considering revascularization procedure. In hibernating myocardium, the stress echocardiography shows a characteristic biphasic response to stimulation (by stress), whereby ventricular function improves at a low level of inotrophic stimulation but subsequently deteriorates at a high level of stimulation. This test can predict which patients may experience improvement in left ventricular function following a revascularization procedure.

SCANNING

Q: What is the role of the computed axial tomography (CAT) scan in the investigation of coronary heart disease?
Computed axial tomography scanning (CAT scan) enables the study of various structures of the heart. Diagnosis of many heart diseases including coronary heart disease can be confirmed. The CAT scan (with contrast enhancement) is widely used for the noninvasive diagnosis of aortic dissection, assessment of pericardial thickness, and the diagnosis of cardiac tumors. Spiral computed tomography (CT) images utilize newer technology that enables more rapid image acquisition, often during a single breath-hold period, at relatively low radiation doses than conventional CT. Electron beam computed tomography (EBCT) or ultrafast CT scan uses a direct electron beam to acquire images in a matter of milliseconds, and

these images can be recorded in a cine motion picture format. EBCT is also used in the investigation of coronary artery disease by virtue of its ability to detect calcification. Additional uses of ultrafast CT include the evaluation of graft patency following coronary bypass surgery, analysis of ventricular wall motion, and blood flow quantification in congenital heart disease, permitting dynamic assessment of shunts and other defects. Noncontrast CT can quantify the site and magnitude of calcium, which is a component of culprit lesions. Potentially, CT of the coronary arteries can provide essential information about the architecture of atherosclerotic plaque.

Magnetic Resonance Imaging (MRI)

Q: What is the role of MRI of the coronary artery in the diagnosis of coronary artery disease (CAD)?
Magnetic resonance imaging uses a powerful field to obtain detailed images of internal structures. This technique is based on the magnetic polarity of hydrogen nuclei, which align themselves with an applied magnetic field. It enables the assessment of myocardial structures and function (e.g., ventricular mass and volume, neoplasm, cardiomyopathies, intracardiac thrombus). Presently, the use of fast gradient echo MR sequences (turbo flash) in combination with breath holding has reduced image acquisition time to a single breath hold and enables accurate identification of coronary arteries and their narrowing. In the context of CAD, two techniques are important: magnetic resonance coronary angiography (MR-CA) and contrast-enhanced MRI. Three-dimensional MR-CA is an accurate noninvasive procedure for detecting disease in the proximal and middle coronary artery segments in some patients, especially those with three-vessel and main-stem disease. Coronary MRI can also detect congenital abnormalities of coronary arteries. Images of the origins and proximal portions of the main coronary arteries and bifurcations are possible but more distal portions are less reliably seen.[4] Coronary artery blood flow and flow reserve can also be measured with MRI using current techniques. Such measurements in the left anterior descending artery or one of its diagonal branches have been shown to correlate well with Doppler velocity-flow measurements at cardiac catheterization.

In contrast-enhanced MRI, a gadolinium-based agent is given intravenously to assess myocardial viability. This substance can penetrate and concentrate in nonviable infarcted areas, appearing "hyperenhanced" as compared to viable. This can help in detecting patients appropriate for revascularization procedures. Given intra-venously, gadolinium redistributes into the tissues. Early imaging shows the enhancement of normal myocardium with darker areas of infarction due to poor perfusion. Conversely, images taken 15 to 20 minutes after gadolinium washout from normal tissues show accumulation in the extracellular water of a myocardial scar, making old infarctions appear bright. A scar of >50% of myocardial wall thickness has a reduced chance of functional recovery after revascularization.[5] High-resolution multicontrast MRI is currently the leading imaging modality for plaque characterization in vivo. It can differentiate a plaque component based on both physical and chemical variables.[6]

NUCLEAR IMAGING

Nuclear imaging may be used to detect MI and to measure myocardial function, perfusion, or viability depending on the radiopharmaceutical used and the technique of imaging. These data are more valuable when used in combination. The gamma camera produces a planer image in which structures are superimposed as in a routine x-ray. Single photon emission computed tomography (SPECT) imaging uses similar raw data to construct tomographic images, just as a CT x-ray constructs images. These methods may be used with any radiopharmaceutical drug.

Q: How is myocardial perfusion imaging performed and what are its strengths and weaknesses?

Myocardial perfusion imaging/scintigraphy (MPI/MPS, thallium scan, radionuclide perfusion imaging) is the only noninvasive method of assessing myocardial perfusion. It can be performed using thallium-201 or technetium-99m, and is useful in assessing myocardial function, ventricular function, myocardial viability, and prognosis. It is the test of choice for patients who cannot manage a treadmill. It is expensive and involves radiation exposure, and the image quality can be attenuated by breast shadows in women. In the diagnosis of CAD, it has a sensitivity of 91% and a specificity of 89%. This is in contrast to exercise testing, which has a sensitivity of 68% and a specificity of 77%.[7] MPI also provides prognostic information, which is more reliable than either treadmill testing or coronary angiography.[8] Moreover, unlike exercise testing it is able to provide more objective evidence of the extent and the size of the myocardial insult. A radioactive substance, usually thallium-201, is injected intravenously while the patient is exercising. Thallium behaves like potassium. Depending on the isotope used, it gets bound to the myocardium or red blood cells. The intracellular concentration of thallium, estimated by the image density, depends on blood supply (perfusion) and membrane function (tissue viability). The radiation then emitted is detected by a gamma camera placed on the chest (Fig. 5.1). In a normal heart, the radionuclide produces a homogeneous distribution of thallium in myocardial tissue. However, the areas that are scarred (by previous infarction) or have reduced perfusion during exercise (i.e. myocardial ischemia) show as light or "cold spots" due to a lower concentration of thallium.

When assessing myocardial ischemia, the initial pictures are taken immediately after exercise, and delayed images are taken 3 to 4 hours later. By then all visible myocytes should have an equal

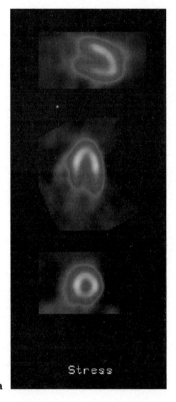

a

FIGURE 5.1. A thallium scan. (a) Normal thallium. (b) Thallium-reversible ischemia in left anterior descending (LAD) territory. (See also color insert.) Reproduced by permission of Dr Arvind Vasudeva, Consultant Cardiologist, Kingston Hospital, Surrey, U.K.

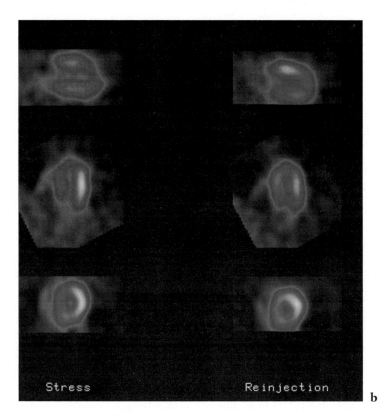

Stress   Reinjection

b

FIGURE 5.1. *Continued.*

concentration of thallium. Any defect due to myocardial ischemia on the initial images should now show a uniform concentration of isotope, representing reversible defect while infracted or scarred tissue remains devoid of thallium, still appearing as a "cold spot." Occasionally, this appearance is also seen in ischemic noncontractile but metabolically active areas, which can regain function if the blood flow is restored. This may occur in hibernating myocardium. Repeat imaging after another thallium injection at rest to increase uptake by viable cells can help differentiate the appearance from that of irreversible scarred tissue. Resting injection of thallium with late reimaging is a sensitive test for assessing myocardial viability. If thallium uptake is more than 50% of normal in infarcted area, then the revascularization procedure is useful. Thus, this procedure is helpful in detecting CAD patients who are likely to respond to the revascularization procedure.

The exercise bicycle is used to produce stress, which reduces the uptake of isotope by the intestine and also improves image quality. However, for those patients who are unable to exercise due to various medical conditions, an artificial state of stress is produced by giving drugs such as adenosine, dobutamine, or dipyridamole. Since dipyridamole produces greater dilatation of normal coronary arteries as compared to atheromatous artery, this produces "coronary steal" phenomenon, where more blood flows in normal coronary arteries but at the expense of diseased ones. This creates a perfusion defect on the thallium scan.

Instead of thallium-201, technetium-99m–labeled compounds (^{99m}Tc-sestamibi [MIBI]) can be used.

Caution
Treadmill testing should always precede the thallium scan, unless there are reasons for not doing so. Thallium testing should not be used as a screening procedure.

Strengths and Weaknesses
Thallium scanning is of little value in determining the number of vessels with significant coronary disease. However, this may be the procedure of choice in the following situations:

- Those patients who have abnormal resting ECG (left bundle branch block [LBBB] or right bundle branch block [RBBB]).
- In patients with past history of MI or revascularization procedure.
- A preferred test where there is single-vessel coronary artery disease.
- Assessment of reversible ischemia.

Thallium scanning does not exclude CAD with certainty, but it is useful in patients who have demonstrated CAD angiographically because if these patients have a normal thallium test, it is indicative of good prognosis. It helps to achieve risk stratification after MI.

If the result of a treadmill test is equivocal, the thallium scan is a useful adjuvant, especially for women in whom false-positive exercise ECGs are common. This is also useful when resting ECG is abnormal, when findings on exercise ECG are equivocal, or when only submaximal exercise has been achieved.

These multiple planar procedures have now been replaced by SPECT imaging, a three-dimensional imaging technique that provides more accurate localization of perfusion defects. Technetium-labeled methoxy isobutyl isonitrile or technetium-labeled tetrofosmin is used. A normal perfusion test even in the presence of angiographically proved cases, predicts a risk of myocardial infarction or cardiac death of less than 1% per year.[9,10]

Q: How is myocardial viability assessed?

Hibernating myocardium occurs with severe and prolonged ischemia accompanied by a reduction of myocardial contraction as a mechanism of myocardium protection, where the metabolism has changed to accommodate itself to hypoxic conditions. Thus, myocytes "sleep" but remain viable. The irreversible damage has not occurred and ventricular function can be improved by surgical revascularization. Myocardial scar refers to the final necrotic lesion. The myocardial viability can be assessed with the following techniques:

- Positron emission tomography (PET).
- ^{201}TI single photon emission computed tomography (TI-SPECT).
- Dobutamine stress echocardiography.
- Myocardial contrast echocardiography (MCE).

Positron Emission Tomography

Positron emission tomography (PET) is the most useful noninvasive nuclear imaging technique in evaluating myocardial ischemia and myocardial viability. It enables the study of coronary blood flow and myocardial metabolism. It usually employs positron-emitting isotopes attached to a metabolic tracer (e.g., rubidium-82, nitrogen-13). Sensitivity detectors then measure positron emission from the tracer molecule. Myocardial perfusion is usually assessed by using nitrogen-13–labeled ammonia or rubidium-82. These flow tracers are taken up by myocytes in proportion to blood flow. Myocardial viability is assessed by combined results of glucose utilization by myocardial tissue and myocardial perfusion. In a normal myocardium, glucose provides about 20% of energy production and the rest is derived from fatty acids. However, in myocardial ischemia more glucose is utilized. Glucose uptake is measured by using fluoro-18-deoxyglucose (FDG). The results of myocardial perfusion and glucose uptake obtained by PET can differentiate among normal myocardium (preserved contractility and positive FDG uptake), infarcted myocardium (impaired contractility and no FDG uptake), and hibernating myocardium (impaired contractility and positive FDG uptake).

CORONARY ANGIOGRAPHY

Q: What are the indications for and pitfalls of coronary angiography?
Coronary angiography provides valuable information in risk stratification and is the most important diagnostic tool in coronary artery disease and in the assessment of suitability for the revascularization procedure. With the aid of this test the severity of anatomical lesions can be assessed, but it is unable to provide any useful information about myocardial perfusion, due to collateral circulation (Fig. 5.2).

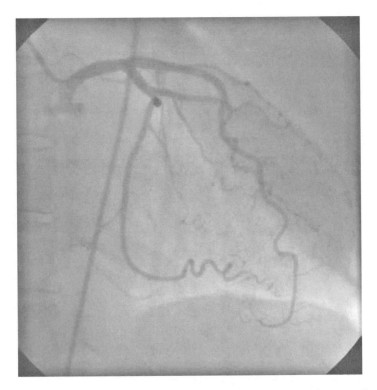

FIGURE 5.2. Coronary angiography. Reproduced by permission of Dr Arvind Vasudeva, Consultant Cardiologist, Kingston Hospital, Surrey, U.K.

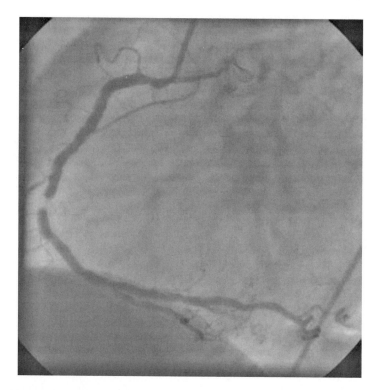

FIGURE 5.2. *Continued.*

Strictly speaking coronary angiography does not diagnose either coronary atheroma (since vessel wall disease may be present when the lumen is normal) or myocardial ischemia (since it does not give full information about coronary flow). This is a simple procedure that can be carried out on an outpatient basis. There is 1 in 2000 risk of nonfatal heart attack and 1 in 1000 risk of nonfatal stroke. During angiography, the tip of the catheter may accidentally dissect the plaque on entry into the left coronary ostium or may completely occlude the already stenosed vessel.

Important indications of coronary angiography are as follows:

- To confirm the diagnosis of angina, when anginal symptoms are not controlled with drugs, or symptoms recur after a revascularization procedure.
- Class I and II stable angina with positive stress test or class III and class IV angina without a positive stress test.
- Unstable angina or non–Q-wave MI following stabilization.
- Severe ventricular arrhythmia.
- Acute myocardial infarction.
- To decide if surgery is indicated in a patient suffering from stable angina where symptoms are significantly affecting the patient's lifestyle.

Pitfalls of Coronary Angiography

Anatomical anomalies of origin and bifurcation of the left coronary artery (LCA) can sometimes give the wrong diagnosis, for instance, if the LCA is absent and instead there are two ostia in the left aortic sinus, one for the LCA and the other for the circumflex artery. During catheterization, the catheter tip may pass into either of these, giving the wrong impression that the other artery is completely blocked. Catheter-induced spasm of the right coronary artery should be distinguished from pathological lesions. Sometimes osteal stenosis of the LCA may not be detected due to a procedural problem.

During catheterization, the radiopaque dye is forced through the arterial tree, and artifactual flow patterns or accentuated filling of branch vessels and collateral circulation may result. The degree to which this occurs largely depends on the size of the artery and the force with which the contrast is injected. Therefore, the degree of opacification of distal branches and the extent to which the collaterals are filled may not reflect the norm. Due to anatomical anomalies, it is possible for occlusions at branch origins to go undetected. In some cases obstruction of a branch can be detected only by late filling of the distant segment of the branch through collateral circulation.

Myocardial bridging is the state in which a short segment of the LCA passes through the myocardium, while the rest takes the normal route (i.e., over the epicardial surface of the heart). This short segment of the LCA has a "bridge" of myocardial fibers passing over it. During systole it gives an erroneous impression that there is atheromatous plaque at that site. A narrow segment seen on the angiogram is usually considered to be a "stenotic area," which may be indistinguishable from a recanalized artery. Angiography is also sometimes unable to detect severe atherosclerotic lesions of the coronary arteries due to vascular remodeling.

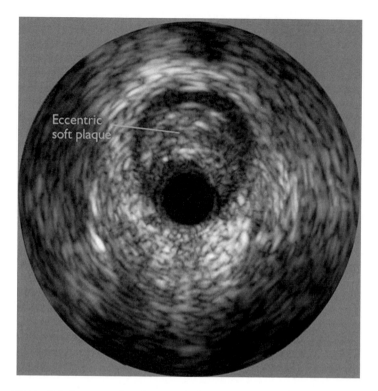

FIGURE 5.3. Intravascular ultrasound showing eccentric plaque.
Reproduced by permission of Dr Arvind Vasudeva, Consultant Cardiologist,
Kingston Hospital, Surrey, U.K.

Intravascular Ultrasound

Intravascular ultrasound (IVUS) provides a cross-sectional, three-dimensional image of the full circumference of the coronary artery (Fig. 5.3). It enables exact measurement of plaque length, thickness, and lumen diameter. It can help to diagnose atherosclerotic plaques, which are otherwise not detected by coronary angiography due to vascular remodeling. IVUS is also used to assess ambiguous angiographic findings and to identify wall dissection or thrombus.

References

1. Weissler AM. Assessment and use of cardiovascular tests in clinical prediction. In: Guiliani ER, Holmes DR, Hayes DL, et al., eds. Mayo Clinic Practice of Cardiology, 3rd ed. St. Louis: Mosby Yearbook, 1996:400.

2. Mickley H. Ambulatory ST segment monitoring after myocardial infarction. Br Heart J 1994;71:113–114.

3. Gibbons RJ, Antman EA, Alpert J, et al. ACC/AHA 2002 guideline update for exercise testing. American College of Cardiology. Circulation 2002;106:1883–1892.

4. Fayed ZA, Fuster V, Fallon JT, et al. Non-invasive in vivo human coronary artery lumen and wall imaging using black-blood magnetic resonance imaging. Circulation 2000;102:506–510.

5. Kim RJ, Fieno DS, Parrish RB, et al. Relationship of MRI delayed contrast enhancement to irreversible injury, infarct age, contractile function. Circulation 1999;100:185–192.

6. Fayed ZA, Fuster V. Clinical imaging of the high-risk or vulnerable atherosclerotic plaque. Circulation 2001;104:249–252.

7. Gianrossi R, Detrano R, Mulvihill D, et al. Exercise induced ST segment depression in the diagnosis of coronary heart disease: a meta-analysis. Circulation 1989;80:87–98.

8. Kaul S, Finnelstein DM, Homma S, et al. Superiority of quantitative exercise thallium-201 variables in determent long-term prognosis in ambulatory patients with chest pain: Comparison with cardiac catheterization. J Am Coll Cardiol 1988;12:25–34.

9. Zaret BL, Wackers FJ. Nuclear cardiology, part 1. N Engl J Med 1993;329:775–783.

10. Zaret BL, Wackers FJ. Nuclear cardiology, part 2. N Engl J Med 1993;329:855–863.

Chapter 6
Coronary Artery Disease

Coronary heart disease (CHD) refers to the consequences of coronary artery disease. It is increasingly common and is the largest single cause of death in the developed world. It is responsible for about 30% of total mortality.

NORMAL STATUS

Q: What is the anatomy of the coronary arteries?
The right coronary artery (RCA) arises from the right coronary sinus, at the base of the aorta. It runs forward in the atrioventricular groove and supplies the sinus node through small branches. It runs downward and around the inferior margin of the heart, giving off a marginal branch that supplies the right ventricular wall. It then descends as the posterior descending artery and supplies the ventricles and interventricular septum. Branches of the RCA supply the conducting tissues, the right ventricle, and the inferior surface of the left ventricular wall.

The left coronary artery (LCA) arises from the left posterior sinus at the base of the aorta. It runs forward between the pulmonary trunk and left atrium to the atrioventricular groove, where it divides into the left anterior descending (LAD) artery and the circumflex artery. The anterior descending artery travels downward in the anterior ventricular groove toward the cardiac apex where it turns around and ascends to anastomose with a posterior ventricular branch of the RCA. During its descent on the anterior surface, the LAD artery gives off septal and diagonal branches. Septal branches supply the anterior two thirds of the interventricular septum and the apical portion of the anterior papillary muscle. Diagonal branches supply the anterior ventricular wall. The left circumflex branch runs round the left margin of the heart in the atrioventricular groove, supplying branches to the left atrium and left surface of the heart. Sometimes the circumflex artery gives rise to the posterior descending artery.

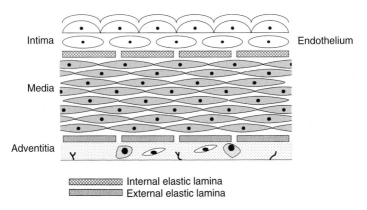

Internal elastic lamina
External elastic lamina

FIGURE 6.1. A schematic diagram of the arterial wall.

Q: What is the structure of the coronary artery and what are its functions?

The normal arterial wall is composed of three layers: intima, media, and adventitia (Fig. 6.1). The intima is composed of two layers: a single thickness of endothelial cells, joined to a basement membrane of proteins, called proteoglycan. The transparent endothelial cells are coated with a glycocalyx, which is made up of free polysaccharides, glycosaminoglycans, and glycoprotein and glycolipid side chains. The glycocalyx is in direct contact with blood circulation and it constitutes an important link between blood and tissues. The function of endothelium tissue is complex but the important ones are the following:

- Provides nonthrombogenic surface (produces antithrombotic molecules)
- Inhibits platelet aggregation and thrombus formation
- Regulates the passage of substances in and out of the arterial wall

Endothelium is selectively permeable to all proteins in the blood. Atherosclerotic changes occur primarily in the intima. The normal intima is of uneven thickness due to a physiologically adaptive thickening at certain sites where the atherosclerotic process is likely to occur. It may develop in utero, or subsequently in healthy individuals. The adaptive thickening may be eccentric (focal) or diffuse (extensive). Eccentric thickening is present at arterial branches and orifices only, and is related to blood turbulence and altered blood flow. This type of change may occur in the aorta, and the coronary, renal, cerebral, and carotid arteries. These (eccentric) areas show increased turnover of endothelial cells, smooth muscle cells (SMCs) and increased concentration of low-density lipoprotein (LDL) and other plasma components. The diffuse thickening is widespread, and may coexist with the eccentric type.

The media is the thickest layer of the arterial wall, composed entirely of SMCs, bounded by internal and external elastic laminae. The laminae contain openings in the elastic layers through which cells can pass. The internal elastic lamina lies between the intima and the media, and is considered part of the media. Arterial dilatation and aneurysm formation occur due to secondary changes in the media caused by atherosclerosis, called vascular remodeling. The external elastic lamina, made of elastic fibers, is situated between the media and the adventitia. The adventitia is composed of fibroblast with sparse SMCs in loose connective tissue. The adventitia contains blood supply in the form of vasa vasorum or capillaries, venules, and arterioles. Nerve fibers and lymphatic channels are also distributed within this layer.

ATHEROGENESIS

Q: What is the pathogenesis of atherosclerosis?
Coronary artery disease (CAD) is a condition characterized by the development of atherosclerotic plaques (fibro-fatty deposits) in the coronary arteries. Atherosclerosis is a chronic and widespread immunoinflammatory disease of large and medium-sized arteries fueled by atherogenic lipoproteins, in particular modified LDL.

Atherosclerosis consists of the formation of fibro-fatty and fibrous lesions, preceded and accompanied by inflammation.[1] Recent advances in basic science have established a fundamental role for inflammation (and underlying cellular and molecular mechanisms) in mediating all stages of this disease from initiation through progression and ultimately the thrombotic complications of atherosclerosis. Despite considerable research, the pathogenesis and complex mechanism of its development remains only partially understood. This is particularly true with the initiating factors. The lesions are the result of various stimuli and healing responses of the arterial wall. This intricate, normally protective process, results from an extremely inflammatory, fibroproliferative response to injury occurring in a hyperlipidemic environment. The atherosclerotic lesions could be classified as types I to VI, which range from minimal intimal change to changes associated with clinical manifestations (Table 6.1).

TABLE 6.1. Stary's classification of atherosclerosis lesions[2]

Type I	Isolated macrophage foam cells, no tissue injury
Type II	Fatty streak, foam cells lipid-laden smooth muscle cells under an intact endothelium
Type III	Type II lesions with increased extra cellular lipid and small lipid pool, microscopic evidence of tissue injury (preatheroma)
Type IV	Extensive lipid core, massive structural injury (atheroma)
Type V	Increased smooth muscle and collagen (fibroatheroma) Va, multiple lipid core; Vb, calcific; Vc, fibrotic
Type VI	Thrombosis or hematoma VIa, disruption of surface; VIb, hematoma; VIc, thrombosis

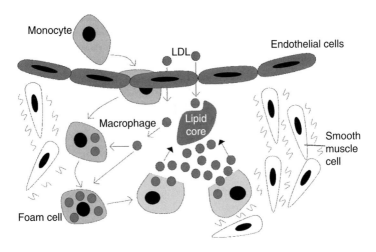

FIGURE 6.2. The process of atherosclerotic plaque formation.
Adapted with permission from: Davies MJ. Pathology and morphology of atherosclerosis. Br J Cardiol 1997;4 (suppl 1):s4–s7.

The development of plaque begins with the adhesions of blood monocytes to the intact endothelium (Fig. 6.2).[1,2] Monocytes move into the intima and migrate into the subendothelial layer where they become macrophages and act as scavenger cells. LDL-C moves freely into the intima.[3] While passing through the endothelial cells, LDL-C gets modified. Modified LDL acts as a chemoattractant that accrues circulating monocytes to the vessel wall, and increases endothelial expression of inflammatory mediators (e.g., monocyte colony-stimulating factor [M-CSF], monocyte chemoattractant protein [MCP-1], and leukocyte adhesion molecules). Further modification of the LDL-C by oxidation leads to a form that is taken up by the macrophages using a scavenger receptor. In diabetes, the sustained raised blood sugar causes glycation of LDL-C; as a result LDL-C becomes antigenic and subsequently proinflammatory. The initial lesions (type I) represent the very initial change and are recognized as an increase in the number of initial macrophages and the appearance of isolated macrophages filled with lipid droplets (microphage foam cells [MFCs]).

In the subendothelial space, macrophages ingest oxidized LDL easily and become foam cells (LDL-C is intracellular), forming the first stage of plaque formation the fatty streak (type II). Fatty streaks can be seen in childhood. Type II lesions are composed of layers of MFCs and lipid-laden SMCs under an intact endothelium. This stage is reversible. Fatty streaks may occur as dots less than 1 mm in diameter or streaks 1 to 2 mm wide and up to 1 cm long. They do not project into the arterial lumen or obstruct blood flow. T lymphocytes also arrive in the intima early during the atherosclerotic process but macrophages and SMCs outnumber them. Macrophages are found in the immediate endothelial area, whereas foam cells are present deep in the proteoglycan layer. The lipid content of this fatty streak is mainly cholesterol oleate and cholesterol linoleate.

In the next stage SMCs migrate from the arterial media to the intima. Proliferation of the SMCs within the intima and secretion of collagen tissue by the SMCs occur. Foam cells, activated platelets, and endothelial cells can all produce substances that cause SMC migration and proliferation. Foam cells produce platelet-derived growth factor (PDGF), which promotes the migration of SMCs into the intimal subendothelial space, where they later multiply. Foam cells also produce cytokines and growth factors (e.g., tumor necrosis factor-α [TNF-α], interleukin-1 [IL-1]), fibroblast growth factors, and transforming growth factor-β, which cause SMCs proliferation and activation of leukocytes.

During the next stage (type III, preatheroma), foam cells die and lipid is extruded into the extracellular space. The extracellular lipids (from various dead foam cells) coalesce to form the lipid core (type IV). The formation of lipid core is a key stage in plaque evolution. Lipids increase the arterial wall's thickness but the lumen remains normal. There are, however, indications of massive structural injury. Even these lesions may not manifest clinically and are also not detected by angiography.

The lipid core becomes encapsulated by increasing number of SMCs, which synthesize collagen. Fibrotic plaques may contain a necrotic core of cell debris, due to the toxic effect of oxidized

LDL and the accumulation of oxygen-derived free radicals and hydrolytic enzymes derived from activated macrophages and T cells. The core of the fibrous plaque is very atherogenic. The type V lesions (fibroatheroma) have prominent SMCs and collagen proliferation. Collagen produced by SMCs appear in a larger amount, producing raised fibrolipid (composed of fibrous tissue and lipid) plaque. Calcification may be superimposed. The lipid core of advanced plaques is surrounded by collagen tissue and separated from the lumen of the artery by a fibrous cap containing muscle cells. The core may occupy a high proportion of overall plaque volume or a low proportion with every gradation in between. The lipid core is highly thrombogenic, containing collagen fragments and tissue factor produced by macrophages. Some plaques appear white due to the presence of collagen, whereas others, which contain high lipid amounts, appear yellow. The formation of type VI lesions represent type V lesions with fissure or hematoma and thrombus. Lesions of types IV, V, and VI are sometimes associated with localized dilations of the part of the vascular wall they occupy. Distinct aneurysms are generally associated with type VI lesion.

The raised fibrolipid or advanced plaque is responsible for the manifestation of clinical symptoms. The advanced plaque does not always cause stenosis or become angiographically detectable in the coronary arteries, due to vascular remodeling, in which the arterial wall dilates (forming an aneurysm), leaving the lumen intact. These lesions may progress slowly to such an extent that they encroach on the lumen or become unstable, undergo thrombosis (vide infra), and produce acute symptoms. Even within individuals, and within one coronary artery, there is large variation in plaques.

Most acute coronary symptoms are due to thrombosis in or on an atheromatous plaque. Thrombosis may occur in two ways. First, the endothelium over the plaque undergoes denudation to expose both collagen and von Willebrand factor to the platelets. A single layer of platelet forms (by activity of the Ia/Ib group of receptors), followed by platelet-to-platelet adhesion (via the IIb/IIIa receptor). As a result, platelets adhere to the damaged endothelial site and release PDGF. Most of the thrombi thus formed are small and do not produce clinical symptoms but may cause major thrombi at segments of preexisting stenosis and in diabetic patients.[4] Second, in disruption of the plaque, the cap tears, which allows blood to enter the lipid core and meet the tissue factor and lipid surface. This forms a platelet-rich thrombus within the plaque. The plaque expands, distorts, and projects into the arterial lumen, causing symptoms of unstable angina with microemboli into intramyocardial arteries. Finally, the thrombus completely blocks the arteries.

Each plaque is the site of an intense inflammatory process, giving rise to the presence of C-reactive protein (CRP). Plaques most likely to rupture are those that are angiographically small to medium in size, have large lipid core (>50% of the overall plaque volume), and have a thin fibrous cap, particularly the one composed of a disorganized pattern of the collagen fibrils, a high macrophage density, and a reduced smooth muscle content. The risk of plaque rupture correlates poorly with the degree of stenosis of the vessel, as half of all myocardial infarctions (MIs) occur in arteries that have <50% luminal diameter narrowing. The role of infecting agents, such as *Chlamydia* and *Helicobacter*, in the pathogenesis of atherosclerosis is described elsewhere in this chapter.

Hypotheses About Atherosclerosis

There are several hypotheses but none is fully accepted. The response to inflammation and injury is the interesting one. The principle of this theory is that the risk factors somehow cause endothelial dysfunction, which can elicit a series of cellular interactions that culminates in the lesion of atherosclerosis.[1] Actual desquamative injury or sloughing of endothelial cells occurs later than dysfunction or activation of these cells. Chronic endothelial injury may occur due to shear forces caused by smoking, hypertension, diabetes, increased hemodynamic forces, hyperlipidemia, angiotensin II, catecholamines, and oxidative stress. Injury occurs particularly at bifurcations. As a result of this injury, endothelial cells lose their smoothness and the glycocalyx-thrombodulin layer. Factor XII and platelets initiate clotting. The chemical and physical factors impair endothelial function by causing the following changes:

- Increasing endothelial permeability (i.e. allowing LDL to pass through).
- Releasing inflammatory cytokines.
- Increasing transcription of cell-surface adhesion molecules.
- Impairing antithrombotic properties.

Therapy for Atherosclerosis

Lipid-lowering drugs, antiplatelet/antithrombotic agents, and antihypertensives play a crucial role.

Q: What types of cells are involved in atherosclerosis?

Four main types of cells are involved in the atherosclerotic process: endothelial cells, smooth muscle cells, platelets, and monocyte-macrophages.

Endothelial Cells

The healthy endothelium not only mediates endothelium-dependent vasodilatation, but also actively suppresses thrombosis, vascular inflammation, and hypertrophy. Antithrombotic factors are the following:

1. Smoothness of the endothelium
2. Presence of the glycocalyx, a mucopolysaccharide that adheres to endothelium and repels clotting factors and platelets
3. Thrombodulin, a protein bound with endothelial membrane, binds thrombin. Alteration in endothelial function may be an important role. Endothelial cells bind LDL through specific high-affinity receptors and mildly oxidize them so that they are engulfed by macrophages. Therefore, endothelial cells may have a role to play in the initiation of atherosclerosis

Endothelial cells also secrete following vasoconstrictors and vasodilators through various stimuli, but the predominant effect is vasodilatation. However, dysfunctional endothelium produces a reduced amount of vasodilators, so that the balance shifts toward vasoconstriction instead:

- Vasoconstrictors: endothelins, PDGF, endothelium-derived constricting factor.
- Vasodilators: endothelium-derived relaxing factor (EDRF), now called nitric oxide (NO), and prostacyclin (inhibits platelet activation), endothelium-derived hyperpolarizing factor (EDHF).

Endothelial dependent vasodilatation predicts CV events. Acute coronary syndrome (ACS), heart failure, and peripheral vascular disease can be improved by statins, ACE inhibitors, reductions in hyperglycemia, diet, and exercise.

Nitric Oxide and Atherosclerosis

Nitric oxide is an important regulatory molecule in cardiovascular function, maintaining vascular tone. It is synthesized in vascular endothelial cells from the abundant amino acid L-arginine by the enzyme endothelial nitric oxide synthase. NO is an important anti-atherogenic molecule. It reduces platelet and monocyte adhesion to the endothelium, SMC proliferation and migration, and plasminogen activator inhibitor-1 (PAI-1) expression. These changes are important in the early stages of atherosclerosis. Additionally, atherosclerotic plaques damage the endothelium and reduce NO release. Oxidized LDL has been shown to reduce the availability of NO. The rings of atherosclerotic coronary arteries have less NO as compared to that of normal coronary arteries. NO causes vasodilatation; therefore, its deficiency may cause increased total peripheral resistance, a characteristic of essential hypertension. Reduced NO production is an independent predictor of acute coronary events. Endothelial nitric oxide synthase (eNOS) has been identified in platelets, making them produce NO.

Smooth Muscle Cells (SMCs)

Smooth muscle cells play an important role in the reparative and proliferate processes of atherosclerosis. Normally, SMCs are not present in the intima but they invade this layer in atherosclerosis. Substances that stimulate SMC to contract include circulating molecules (e.g., angiotensen II), those released from local nerve terminals (e.g., acetylecholine), and those originating from the overlying endothelium (e.g., endothelin). In healthy blood vessel, SMCs produce collagen, elastin, and proteoglycans that form the vascular extracellular matrix. SMCs can also produce various vasoactive and inflammatory mediators such as cytokines, particularly IL-6 and TNF-α, which can increase lymphocytic proliferation, initiate endothelial expression of leukocyte adhesion molecules, and propagate an inflammatory response.

Platelets

Platelets play a role in atherosclerosis in the following ways:

- Aggregation and adhesion
- Release of mitogenic (cell-division–stimulating, e.g., epidermal growth factor [EGF] and PDGF, which is considered the most potent) and chemotactic (white-blood-cell attracting) factor. PDGF increases collagen proliferation and promotes increased LDL uptake.

Monocytes

Monocytes/macrophages are the scavenger cells. Circulating monocytes are recruited to the intima by the expression of adhesive glycoprotein on the glycocalyx. Adhesive glycoprotein production is believed to be induced by mildly oxidized LDL. With monocyte adhesion to the vessel wall, monocyte chemotactic protein-1 and colony-stimulating factor are secreted, so that more monocytes are attracted to this site. Macrophages possess receptors for native, or natural, LDL and for oxidized LDL. By producing reactive oxygen species, macrophages play a crucial role in atherogenesis. Endothelin also mildly oxidizes LDL. Monocytes also produce the following growth factors:

- PDGF for connective tissue cells, including SMCs and fibroblasts.
- Fibroblast growth factor (FGF) for vascular endothelium.
- EGF for endothelial cells.

Q: What are the complications of atherosclerosis? What are the sequlae of CAD?
The complications of atherosclerosis are initiated at certain sites where fibrous plaque is first likely to be formed. These sites include the dorsal aspect of the abdominal aorta and proximal coronary arteries, followed by popliteal arteries, the descending thoracic aorta, internal carotid arteries, and renal arteries. Fibrous plaque does not affect the whole arterial system uniformly. The complications prone to occur in fibrous plaque include calcification, rupture, hemorrhage, and embolism. The following are the complications of atherosclerosis:

- Calcification of fibrous plaque leads to rigidity of blood vessels. Progression of plaques causes narrowing of the coronary arteries, leading to symptoms of myocardial ischemia. Claudication in the limbs may occur as a result of organization of microthrombi within the lesion.
- Ulceration and rupture of fibrous plaque leads to thrombus formation, causing myocardial ischemia or unstable angina.
- Hemorrhage into the fibrous plaque increases its size.
- Weakening of the vessel wall leads to an aortic aneurysm caused by atrophy of muscle cells, and loss of elastic tissue due to pressure effects.
- Embolization of detached fragments causes emboli in cerebral arteries (e.g., stroke, transient ischemic attack [TIA]) and renal arteries (renal failure).

Sequelae of Coronary Artery Disease (Coronary Events)
Coronary artery disease can remain asymptomatic or cause the following coronary events:

- Angina pectoris (stable or unstable).
- Sudden death.
- Acute myocardial infarction.
- Silent ischemia.
- Arrhythmias.

- Heart failure or left ventricular dysfunction.
- Ischemic cardiomyopathy.

RISK FACTORS

Q: What are the risk factors for coronary heart disease?
The risk factors for CHD may be modifiable (capable of change by some form of intervention) or nonmodifiable. Nonmodifiable factors include male gender, increasing age, ethnic origin, low birth weight, and family history; all other factors are modifiable. The following risk factors can lead to CHD:

- Cigarette smoking.
- High blood pressure (particularly systolic) or those currently taking antihypertensive medication, or high-normal blood pressure.
- Dyslipidemia: raised LDL cholesterol, low HDL-C, and raised triglycerides (especially VLDL remnants and possibly small LDL particles).
- Diabetes, impaired glucose intolerance (impaired fasting glucose is not), metabolic syndrome.
- Age and sex (≥45 for men, ≥55 for women or premature menopause without estrogen replacement) and ethnicity.
- Obesity (BMI ≥30 kg/m²) or abdominal obesity.
- Family history of premature cardiovascular disease.
- Hemostatic and thrombogenic factors: tissue type plasminogen activator (tPA)/PAI-1, thrombin activatable fibrinolysis inhibitor, fibrinogen, D-dimer, factor V Leiden.
- Physical inactivity.
- Personal history of atherosclerosis.
- Markers for inflammation: hsCRP, serum amyloid A, IL-6, IL-18, TNF, cell adhesion molecules, CD40 ligand, myeloperoxidase.[5]
- Nontraditional lipid markers: lipoprotein (a), apoA, apoB, particle size, particle density.[5]
- Markers of oxidation: oxidized LDL (and antibodies against oxidized LDL), glutathione.[5]
- Others: estrogen, left ventricular hypertrophy, erectile dysfunction, microalbuminuria, psychosocial factors, low birth weight, hyperhomocystinemia.

In order of importance, the four most important risk factors are dyslipidemia, hypertension, cigarette smoking, and increasing age. Obesity, family history of premature CHD, and physical inactivity contribute to other risk factors and are now major risk factors in their own right.

Family History

A family history risk entails premature CHD or other atherosclerotic disease in a male first-degree relative before the age of 55 years, or in a female first-degree relative before the age of 65 years. A family history of MI is an independent risk factor for CHD. This risk may be due to genetic factors or the effect of a shared environment (diet, smoking, etc.). It is estimated that about 40% of the risk of developing ischemic heart disease is controlled by genetic factors, and 60% by environmental factors. Hyperlipidemia, hyperfibrinogenemia, and abnormalities of other coagulation factors are often genetically determined. A positive family history increases the risk by a factor of approximately 1.5 and should also be taken into account in assessing individual risk. Risk rises further if more than one family member is affected. A history of heart attack in two or more first-degree relatives triples the risk of CHD. There is an increased rate of CHD in the siblings of affected twins, although that effect diminishes with age.

Age and Sex

As atheroma occurs gradually over many years, age becomes an important factor. CHD is rare in young men 20 to 30 years of age and young women 20 to 40 years of age, except in those with severe risk factors (e.g., familial hypercholesterolemia, heavy cigarette smoking, or diabetes). Therefore, risk factors should be identified at a young age. Most new CHD events and most coronary deaths occur in older people (≥65 years). Middle-aged men from 35 to 65 have a higher CHD risk than women, because they have a high prevalence of risk factors, and are predisposed to abdominal obesity and the metabolic syndrome. In women between the ages of 45 to 75, the onset of CHD is delayed by some 10 to 15 years compared to men; thus most CHD in women occurs after age 65 years. Most deaths due to CHD in women under the age of 65 years occur due to multiple risk factors and the metabolic syndrome.

Ethnicity

CHD is more common among South Asians (of the Indian subcontinent), but less common in African Caribbeans. Stroke is much more common in the latter group than in Caucasians. South Asian descent entails a 40% greater risk of CHD. Among Asians an increased rate of CHD appears to be related to diabetes and insulin resistance, whereas African Caribbeans have reduced risk due to low insulin resistance. In the United States, African Americans have the highest overall CHD mortality rates, the reason for which is not clear, but other factors (e.g., high blood pressure, left ventricular failure, diabetes mellitus, smoking, obesity, physical inactivity) play a role. For West Africans the rate of stroke is nearly three times higher for men and 81% higher for women. For Caribbeans it is 68% higher for men and 57% higher for women. Japan, despite a high rate of smoking, has a very low CHD rate, which is paralleled by equally low average serum cholesterol. The exact opposite is the case in Finland.

Hemostatic and Thrombogenic Factors

Hemostatic factors associated with increased risk of coronary events include increased level of fibrinogen, activator factor VII, PAI-1, tPA, von Willebrand factor, factor V Leiden, and decreased antithrombin III. A low fibrinogen level indicates reduced risk. An elevated plasma level of tPA is apparently associated with increased MI and stroke in healthy men. Fibrinogen increases blood viscosity and platelet aggregation, leading to a hypercoagulable state, promoting thrombosis. It also plays an important role in atherogenesis by fibrin deposition in vessel walls and may promote SMC migration and proliferation. Fibrinogen levels are increased in smoking, sedentary lifestyle, increased triglycerides, hypercholesterolemia, obesity, advancing age, oral contraceptive pills use, and stress. A raised level of activated factor VII is associated with an increased incidence of CHD. Plasminogen activator inhibitor-1 plays an important role in clotting. Elevated concentrations of PAI-1 are associated with an increased risk of recurrent heart attack, and higher levels have been seen in patients with unstable angina and insulin-resistant states. Adult Treatment Panel (ATP) 111 does not recommend measurement of prothrombotic factors as part of the routine assessment of CHD risk.

Inflammation-Sensitive Plasma Proteins (ISP)

All ISPs are associated with the incidence of cardiovascular disease, with largely the same relative risk for all individual ISPs (fibrinogen, orosomucoid, α_1-antitrypsin, haptoglobin, and ceruloplasmin).[6] Studies have reported that the relationship between elevated ISPs and an increase incidence of acute coronary event is now well established. One study showed that men who have been exposed to low-grade inflammation many years earlier have higher fatality in future acute coronary events, with a high proportion of CHD death and less nonfatal MI.[6]

Hormone Replacement Therapy

Hormone replacement therapy (HRT) has not been shown to be beneficial in preventing CHD in women both with and without a previous history of CHD. In fact, studies have shown a slight tendency to increased the rate of CHD in 1 to 2 years of treatment with HRT. Estrogen favorably influences lipid and lipoprotein level, but this did not translate into a reduction of CHD risk in the Heart and Estrogen/Progestin Replacement Study (HERS) study.[7] Two important published controlled studies have failed to confirm a beneficial effect of HRT on cardiovascular disease. The HERS was designed to test the hypothesis that treatment with estrogen 0.625 mg/d with progestin would reduce the combined incidence of nonfatal MI and CHD death compared with a placebo in women with a prior history of heart attack, coronary revascularization, or angiographic evidence of CHD. This was the first large-scale randomized clinical-outcome trial of HRT for the prevention of CHD in postmenopausal women. After an average of 4.1 years of follow-up, there was no difference in the primary outcome of nonfatal heart attack and coronary death between the hormone and placebo arms. Numerous explanations have been proposed for the overall null effect of HRT in HERS. These include inadequate duration of follow-up, adverse effects of medroxyprogesterone acetate, bidirectional effects of estrogen (early risk and late benefit), a population of women too old to benefit from therapy (average age was 66.7 years), a preparation of HRT that was not ideal, chance, or the possibility that HRT is ineffective in preventing recurrent cardiovascular events in women with established disease. Similarly, The Women's Health Initiative (2002) has reported no benefit with HRT on the progression of cardiovascular disease.[8] Therefore, HRT should not be initiated in postmenopausal women with CHD for the purpose of reducing CHD, but if a woman has been on HRT for some time, she could continue with the expectation that there may be some late benefit.

Erectile Dysfunction

Erectile dysfunction (ED) is thought to be a marker for CHD. It is estimated that between 39% and 64% of males with cardiovascular disease (CVD) suffer from erectile dysfunction. Erectile dysfunction can be associated with atherosclerosis, CAD, hypertension, and peripheral vascular disease. The Massachusetts Male Aging Study found that after age adjustment, men with heart disease, diabetes, or hypertension are four times more likely to develop some degree of ED compared with men who do not suffer from these disorders; 60.9% of patients with hypertension and

77.9% of patients with both hypertension and diabetes admitted to ED problems.[9]

Erectile Dysfunction in Coronary Artery Disease

Atherosclerosis may affect small penile arteries. A study observed that in a group of healthy men complaining of ED, 60% had abnormal cholesterol levels, and >90% showed evidence of penile arterial disease during Doppler ultrasound imaging (95th Annual Meeting of the American Urology Association 2000, Atlanta).[10] The atherosclerotic process may actually begin in the small penile arteries.[11] The penile arteries are 1 to 2 mm wide, compared to coronary arteries, which are 3 to 4 mm wide. Narrowing and dysfunction in these vessels might suggest problem in other arteries. Therefore, ED can be a sign of more widespread vascular deterioration.

Erectile Dysfunction in Diabetes

There is strong and independent association between ED and silent myocardial ischemia in apparently uncomplicated type 2 diabetes.[12] Therefore, ED can be a potent predictor of silent CAD among diabetic patients. In addition, the high prevalence of ED among patients with silent CAD emphasizes the usefulness of a treadmill test before starting a treatment for ED, especially in patients with additional cardiovascular risk factors. Over 50% of diabetic men have suffered from ED at some stage, and as many as 39% suffer from ED at all times.[13] Atherosclerosis also affects the penile and pudendal arteries, impairing blood supply to the corpus cavernosum. Autonomic neuropathy is a major contributor to ED in diabetic men.

Lipoprotein (a)

A new lipid and lipoprotein fraction, such as small dense LDL particles, apolipoproteins A1 and B, HDL subfractions, and lipoprotein (a), have been associated with CHD risk. Lipoprotein (a) [Lp(a)] is an independent risk factor. Lipoprotein (a) consists of two components: an LDL particle and an attached apolipoprotein (a). A small number of LDL molecules sometimes possess a protein in addition to Apo B. This additional protein is called apolipoprotein (a) [Apo (a)]. With Apo (a) attached to LDL, the whole complex is called Lp (a). The complex structure may explain its athrogenic and thrombogenic properties. Lp (a) has been recognized as a risk factor for CAD when its level is elevated (>30 mg/dl [0.78 mmol/L]) and associated with high LDL-C (>163 mg/dl [>4.22 mmol/L])[14]. Many retrospective and cross-sectional studies suggest a positive association between Lp (a) and vascular risk. Whether it adds prognostic information is not clear. At present there is no randomized trial evidence that lowering Lp (a) lowers vascular risk. Some studies, however, have cast doubt on its independent role as a risk factor, suggesting that Lp (a) synergistically contributes to CAD by potentiating the effect of other lipid risk factors. Lp (a) accumulates at the site of atherosclerotic lesions and has been found in the plaques.[15] If Lp (a) is raised, an antiplatelet agent should be prescribed. The Apo B/Apo A-1 ratio should also be regarded as highly predictive in evaluating cardiac risk.[16]

Psychosocial Factors

The role of stress as a coronary risk factor is controversial, though there is some evidence that stress, such as divorce, bereavement, or unemployment, may be a risk factor, and that stress management may decrease rates of heart attack in people with CHD. Once CAD has developed, there is firm evidence to indicate that stress is deleterious and may provoke ischemic events.[17,18] It is also likely that psychosocial factors such as depression, hostility, and low levels of support can increase the risk of CHD. It is thought that excessive cardiovascular reactivity to psychological stress may provide the psychological link between psychological factors and CHD. Increased heart rate and high blood pressure associated with stress response may increase intimal injury through hemodynamic forces, such as turbulent blood flow and shear stress on the endothelium. Increased sympathetic activity causes coronary artery pressure surges and tone increase, leading to plaque rupture and thrombus formation. Adrenaline and noradrenaline can alter metabolism and permeability of the arterial wall, decreasing oxygen uptake and affecting platelet aggregation and thus promoting the atherosclerotic process. The exact relationship of depression and CHD is not known, but it appears that serotonin in depressed patients promotes thrombogenesis. A program of stress management incorporated within a cardiac rehabilitation program may be beneficial.[19]

Other Risk Factors

Some conditions are markers or predictors of CHD. They include diabetic retinopathy and nephropathy, microalbuminuria, and hypertension with complications. Left ventricular hypertrophy is a strong predictor, only second to age in predictive power. In fact, it is probably the most important predictor of future events. There is also the risk of sudden death due to arrhythmia.

Q: Are noncoronary atherosclerotic diseases predictor of CHD?

There is evidence that clinical atherosclerotic disease of non-CAD is a powerful predictor of CHD. Clinical forms of noncoronary atherosclerotic carry a risk for clinical CHD, approximately equal to that of established CHD and therefore constitute a CHD risk equivalent. These include peripheral arterial disease (PAD), carotid artery disease (TIA, stroke, or >50% stenosis on angiography or ultrasound), and abdominal aneurysm (ATP 111). These patients have the same LDL-C goal of <100 mg/dL (2.6 mmol/L). High CHD event rates have been seen in asymptomatic patients with advanced carotid artery stenosis. Some studies have suggested that carotid intimal-medial thickening (carotid narrowing <50%) in an asymptomatic patient is associated with increased risk for CHD.

Stroke and MI share common risk factors. The long-term risk of CHD in stroke patients, however, is at least twofold that of age-matched controls in most studies. There is a case for looking for CHD in a patient with carotid stenosis. Data from the Framingham study[20] indicate a higher risk of MI and vascular death in a patient with a carotid bruit compared with those without a bruit. In fact, both a bruit and the degree of stenosis indicated higher cardiovascular risk. The evidence suggest that the ischemic stroke subtype provides important information on concomitant cardiac risk especially in three situations:

- Small vessel cause of stroke (lower risk).
- Significant symptomatic carotid stenosis (higher risk).
- Cardiac embolism as the suspected cause of stroke (very high risk).

The total cholesterol/HDL ratio and CRP are the strongest independent predictors of development of peripheral arterial disease; then comes high-sensitivity (hs)CRP, interleukin-6, soluble intercellular adhesion molecule-1 (sICAM-1), and finally fibrinogen.[21]

Progressive narrowing of arteries in lower extremities due to atherosclerosis causes PAD. Major risk factors for PAD include hypertension, hypercholesterolemia, diabetes, smoking, and low kidney function. There is a positive association between PAD and inflammatory markers, including CRP and fibrinogen.

Q: What is the association between inflammatory markers and atherosclerosis? How can they help in the stratification of CHD risk factors?

Inflammation occurs in the vascular tree as a response to injury, lipid peroxide, and perhaps infection. An inflammatory process not only promotes initiation and progression of atheroma but also contributes to precipitating thrombotic complications of atheroma. Various harmful agents such as smoking, hypertension, and diabetes may play an important role in initiating chronic inflammation, which predisposes vulnerable plaque to rupture and thrombosis. Some of the inflammatory markers for CHD are as follows:

- Inflammatory mediators: raised proinflammatory cytokines (e.g., IL-1β, IL-6, IL-8, TNF-α, and interferon-γ (IFN-γ), increased monocyte adhesion molecules (e.g., sICAM-1), soluble vascular circulating adhesion molecule [sVCAM-1] and E-selectin) and activated nuclear factor-kappa B (NF-κB).
- Acute phase proteins: high levels of CRP, serum amyloid A-protein, and fibrinogen.
- Miscellaneous: raised erythrocyte sedimentation rate (ESR), increased white blood cells, reduced serum albumen.

The process of atherosclerosis is mediated largely by cellular adhesion molecules (CAMs). The evidence for this comes from several sources such as that atherosclerotic plaques contain many CAMs, and CRP induces expression of CAMs in endothelial cells. This is important since cytokines involved in the inflammatory process, such as IL-6 and TNF, stimulate production of CAMs and CRP. The inflammatory cells, together with altered endothelial cells, secrete proinflammatory cytokines, growth factors, leukocyte chemoattractants, adhesion molecules, and collagen-degrading metalloproteinases. This reduces the integrity of the plaque cap, potentially initially an acute event. As atherosclerosis is a generalized disease, and plaques are multiple, sufficient inflammatory markers are produced to enable their measurement in laboratory. Cytokines (e.g., IL-6) move to the liver and increase production of CRP and serum amyloid A (SAA). Elevated CRP levels are a marker of increased production of IL-1 and IL-6. CRP itself can activate monocytes to produce tissue factor, activate complement, and induce monocytes and endothelial release of IL-1 and IL-6. The latter two cytokines are prothrombotic. There is now considerable evidence that an increased level of inflammatory markers, especially hsCRP, in blood indicate higher cardiovascular risk and in acute coronary syndrome predict an unfavorable outcome, independent of the severity of the atherosclerotic lesion or myocardial damage.

C-reactive protein is a reliable measure of underlying systemic inflammation and a strong independent predictor of future MI, stroke, PAD, and sudden cardiac death, even in apparently healthy individuals.[22] In several studies, hsCRP has been shown to add prognostic information at all levels of LDL-C and at all levels of risk as determined by the Framingham Risk Score.[23] Recently, the American Heart Association (AHA) and the Centers for Disease Control and Prevention issued clinical guidelines for the use of hsCRP and suggested that evaluation be considered for those deemed by global risk prediction to be at intermediate risk. It is suggested that the level of CRP also indicates the severity of cardiovascular risk. The AHA has recommended that CRP values be stratified as follows: <1 mg/L indicates low risk, 1 to 3 mg/L indicates moderate risk, >3 mg/L indicates high risk, and 10 to 100 mg/L is suggestive of acute phase response, which should be ignored and repeated in 3 weeks.[24] CRP is composed of five 23-kd subunits. It is a circulating pentraxin that plays a major role in the human innate immune response.[25] CRP in the high normal range has been found to be a potent predictor of future vascular events. The lowest elevation of CRP is noticed in most cardiac cases. The moderate elevation is seen in stable plaques and greater elevation in ruptured plaques. The association of CRP and CVD has been shown in the Physician's Health Study.[26] In this study, physicians in the highest quartile of hsCRP at baseline had a twofold higher risk of stroke, a threefold higher risk of MI, and a fourfold higher risk of PAD. Moreover, the risk associated with hsCRP was independent of other CHD risk factors. In fact, it is possible that CRP, besides being a marker, may also participate as a mediator in atherosclerosis. Cigarette smoking is associated with high levels of CRP.

Four inflammatory markers (hsCRP, SAA, IL-6, and sICAM) were found to be significant predictors of risk, with the hsCRP level outperforming homocysteine, lipoprotein (a), and LDL-C.[26] Men who have been exposed to a low-grade inflammation many years earlier have higher mortality in future coronary events, with a higher proportion of CHD deaths and less nonfatal MI. This relation should be noted when inflammation markers are considered for risk assessment in primary prevention.[6] Moreover, certain treatments that reduce coronary risk also reduce inflammation. There is no evidence as yet that lowering CRP reduces vascular risk. Cell adhesion molecules can be measured in the peripheral blood as a soluble molecule (sCAMs), which are found to be predictive of ischemic events in healthy men.[26] The levels of soluble CAMs have been shown to be elevated in acute coronary syndrome and to predict events in patients with stable angina.[27]

Enzyme cyclooxygene (COX) exists in two isoforms, COX-1 and COX-2, and plays an important role in inflammation. COX-2 may contribute to early atherosclerosis. The selective inhibitor of COX-2 therefore may have an antiinflammatory effect.[28] Aspirin has been shown to reduce the risk of cardiovascular events as much as 44%. The benefit of aspirin in primary prevention is more marked when CRP is very high, and the benefit declines in direct relation with

CRP levels, suggesting that the benefit of aspirin in part may be due to antiinflammatory effect.[29]

Dyslipidemia and Inflammation

According to the oxidation theory, LDL-C retained in the intima undergoes oxidative modification. These modified lipids can induce the expression of adhesion molecules, chemokines, proinflammatory cytokines, and other mediators of inflammation in macrophages and arterial wall cells. LDL-C oxidation theory, however, remains unproven. Lipoproteins such as VLDL and intermediate-density lipoprotein (IDL) also have considerable atherogenic properties. Like LDL, they can also undergo oxidative process. In addition, some evidence suggests that beta-VLDL particles may themselves activate inflammatory function of vascular endothelial cells.[30] Other agents that reduce CRP include lipid-lowering agents, clopidogrel, abciximab, and peroxisome proliferative activator receptor.

Hypertension, Diabetes, and Inflammation

Hypertension follows closely behind lipids on the list of classical risk factors for atherosclerosis. Inflammation may participate in hypertension, providing a pathophysiological link between the two. Angiotensin II can contribute by stimulating the growth of smooth muscles and being a vasoconstrictor can initiate internal inflammation. Like hypertension, inflammation links diabetes to atherosclerosis. Obesity itself causes inflammation and potentiates atherogenesis independently of the effects of insulin resistance and lipoproteins. Elevated CRP has been correlated with both the presence and prognosis of non-ST segment ACS. Elevation of hsCRP depends on the clinical syndrome. Elevated CRP (>3 mg/L) has been observed in <10% normal, <20% of patients with stable angina or variant angina, in >65% of patients with unstable angina (Braunwald class IIIb), in >90% of patients with acute MI (AMI) preceded by unstable angina, and in <50% of those in whom the infarction was totally unheralded (in samples taken before elevation of markers of necrosis).[31,32]

Q: Are microbial agents responsible for coronary heart disease?
It is thought that low-grade inflammatory response is part of atherosclerosis and that bacterial infection plays a crucial role. Infectious agents can furnish inflammatory stimuli that enhance atherosclerosis. However, despite considerable evidence, the direct link between infections (bacterial and viral) and atherosclerosis keeps eluding detection. Infectious agents might also conceivably furnish inflammatory stimuli that accentuate atherogenesis.[32]

Chlamydia when present in the vascular bed can release lipopolysaccharide (endotoxin) and heat shock proteins that can stimulate the production of proinflammatory mediators by vascular endothelial cells and SMCs and infiltrating leukocytes alike.[33] Chronic extravascular infections (e.g., gingivitis, prostatitis, bronchitis, etc.) can increase extravascular production of inflammatory cytokines that may accelerate the evolution of remote atherosclerotic lesions. Many human plaques that show evidence of infections by microbial agents such as *Chlamydia pneumoniae, Helicobacter pylori*, herpes simplex, or cytomegalovirus, predict vascular risk. *C. pneumoniae* is found within plaques, reaches high concentration within macrophages and is rarely found in normal arteries. *C. pneumonae* (Cp) infections, as represented by anti-Cp antibodies in the blood of 220 male MI survivors, were observed to be associated with cardiovascular events over a mean follow-up period of 18 months.[34] Cp antigen has been identified in other vascular beds besides the coronary vessels, such as carotid and peripheral vascular plaques.[35] The data linking *H. pylori* to coronary events, however, is less conclusive. Most previous studies of associations between chronic *H. pylori* infection and CHD have been too small or prone to bias. Viral agents involved include adenovirus, coxsackie virus, and representatives of the herpes viridae. There appears to be an association between high levels of antibodies to enteroviruses, measured by the use of a group-specific antigen, and the risk of MI.[36] Cytomegalovirus is the herpes virus most strongly associated with CHD and atherosclerosis. Herpes simplexvirus-1 (HSV-1) and HSV-2 are found in atherosclerotic lesions. It was demonstrated that high levels of antibodies or circulatory immune complexes against HSV-1 and chlamydia were risk factors for future coronary events in a prospective cohort of middle-aged dyslipidemic men.[36]

Q: What is the role of genes in the development of CHD?

In recent years, the understanding of genetics and molecular medicine has advanced dramatically. Coronary artery disease (CAD) is multifactorial and includes a strong genetic component. Genetic markers are variants in the DNA code (known as alleles) that, alone or in combination, are associated with a specific disease phenotype. Markers with a high predicted value are most useful in clinical medicine. Single nucleotide polymorphisms (SNPs) or variants at a single DNA base pair have received a lot of attention as potential genetic markers.

The disorders that increase the risk of atheroma and thrombus formation are complex processes resulting from genetic and environmental interactions (Table 6.2)[37]. It is well recognized that CAD

TABLE 6.2. Genes responsible for coronary heart disease[37]

Guanine nucleotide binding protein β polypeptide-3
Glucocorticoid receptor
Paraoxonase-1, paraoxonase-2
Nitric oxide synthase-3
Lipoprotein lipase protein
Apolipoprotein B
Angiotensin I converting enzyme-1
Plasminogen activator inhibitor-1
Lipoprotein receptor—related protein
Peroxisome proliferative activated receptor a
Phospholipase A_2 group VII
Interleukin-6
C-reactive protein
Haptoglobin
Hemochromatosis
Angiotensinogen
β-adrenergic receptor
Adducin-1(a)

and AMI run in families because of shared genetic and environmental factors. The evidence for this is as follows:

1. Familial clustering of CAD risk factors: The major risk factors of CAD often show familial clustering that could be due to the effects of shared environmental and inherited factors such as raised lipids and hypertension, both of which predispose to CAD.

2. Inheritance of independent genetic risk factors: A family history of CAD is a strong predictor of CAD, independently of the familial clustering of risk factors. Genetic studies involving twins and well-characterized pedigrees have established that the cardiovascular risk profile indicates a substantial heritable component.

3. Inheritance of susceptibility. The familial clustering of CAD may also be caused by an increased familial susceptibility to the effects of cardiovascular risk factors such as smoking. Susceptibility may be due to various factors such as inherited abnormalities of coagulation. In these patients, the risk of cigarette smoking will be enhanced.

It is clear that genetic factors influence qualitative traits (e.g., levels of LDL-C and HDL-C, blood pressure, adiposity, and left ventricular mass). It is therefore not surprising that the causative basis of complex cardiovascular disorders (e.g., atherothrombosis) involves a dynamic interplay among multiple genes in addition to a gene–environment interaction.[37]

For the development of atherosclerosis, the genes responsible for vessel tone and the response to inflammation and vessel wall damage may be implicated. Elevated circulating factor VII and fibrinogen are indicators for future coronary events. The fibrinolytic inhibitor (activates thrombus formation), PAI-1, has been noted to be raised in young survivors of AMI who developed a recent event. Initial levels of fibrinogen, von Willebrand factor, and tPA are also independent predictors of future acute coronary syndromes. Many of the proteins involved in coagulation and fibrinolysis are under genetic control; therefore, genes could be regarded as risk factors. This theory is further supported by the fact that mutation of the LDL receptor gene leads to familial hypercholesterolemia, which is an autosomal-dominant condition.

In most patients, raised lipids can be caused by both genetic and environmental factors (polygenic or multifactorial hyperlipidemia). In these cases, the genetic effect becomes apparent only in the presence of specific environment factors, such as some variants of the lipoprotein lipase (LPL) gene (the key enzyme of plasma triglyceride metabolism), which appears to increase the risk of developing raised triglycerides, only if a person becomes obese. Recent studies have also implicated common variations of LPL gene in metabolic syndrome. Genetic difference in the nuclear receptor peroxisome proliferator receptor-γ (PPARγ) appears to play a key role in metabolic syndrome. Several of the genes recently identified exhibit common variations that influence CHD risk. The effect of elevated levels of lipoprotein with raised LDL is mediated entirely by genetic factors.

Several studies have supported the genetic role in the pathogenesis of CAD. The angiotensin-converting enzyme (ACE) gene contains an insertion/deletion (I/D) polymorphism, the DD genotype of which has been associated with CAD and MI.

Factor VII

Increased factor VII activity represents a risk factor for ischemic cardiovascular disease. Blood levels of factor VII are influenced by both environmental and genetic factors. Triglycerides are a major determinant of factor VII. The levels of factor VII and their response to environment stimuli is genetically determined. There is a strong association between a common polymorphism of factor VII gene and plasma factor VII levels; however, there was no association between the polymorphins and the risk of ischemic vascular disease. It has been concluded that certain polymorphisms of the factor VII gene may influence the risk of MI, and this effect may be mediated by alterations in factor VII levels.

Thrombomodulin Gene Mutations Associated with Heart Attack
Thrombomodulin is an important receptor for thrombi on the endothelial cell surface of most blood vessels, including those of heart. Thrombin-bound thrombomodulin activated protein C inhibits thrombin generation by degrading factors Va and VIIIa. The finding suggested that mutation in the promoted region of the thrombomodulin gene might constitute a risk for arterial thrombosis. It is observed that in men a variant of prothrombin is associated with an increased risk of MI. The combined presence of major cardiovascular risk factors and a carrier of the coagulation defect increases the risk considerably.

It has been concluded that patients with the small, dense LDL of the atherogenic lipoprotein profile (pattern B) experience a threefold increased risk of CAD, and pattern B is also correlated with the development of type 2 diabetes. A routine lipid profile does not detect the most common inherited dyslipidemias, and in these cases sophisticated tests such as gradient gel electrophoresis can detect disease-relevant lipidemic details (e.g., LDL subclass pattern, LDL particle diameter, and LDL subregions).

The common polymorphism is related to at least two disease entities. First, dysbetalipoproteinemia can affect people with two versions of the Apo E-2 isoform. This rare form of hyperlipidemia increases the risk of atherosclerotic disease. It is more severe when it is caused by mutation in the receptor-binding domain of Apo E. Second, the rate of CHD in patients with Apo E-4 is about 40% higher than the patients with Apo E-3/E-3.

Q: What is the role of antioxidants in coronary heart disease?
Antioxidants include vitamin E (α-tocopherol), vitamin C (ascorbic acid), beta-carotenes, bioflavonoids, and selenium. Evidence of CHD risk reduction from dietary antioxidants is not strong enough to justify the recommendation for antioxidant supplementation to reduce CHD. However, ATP 111 suggests the current recommendation of dietary antioxidants: 75 mg of vitamin C for women and 90 mg for men, and 15 mg of vitamin E. A specific recommendation for beta-carotene was not made.

Evidence from Trials
In the Cambridge Heart Antioxidant Study (CHAOS), a secondary prevention study that used vitamin E in the dose of 400 to 800 IU

daily for 17 months, nonfatal MI was dramatically reduced by 77%, but there was a nonsignificant increase in overall mortality and fatal MI.[38] The Alpha Tocopherol Beta Carotene Cancer Prevention (ATBC) study also did not find any benefit.[39] In fact, the risk of lung cancer in Finnish smokers was increased. The Heart Protection Study, which included 10,000 patients who were given a combination of vitamin E 600 mg, vitamin C 250 mg, and beta-carotene 20 mg, showed no benefit as compared to placebo.[40] No differences existed in the incidence of all-cause or cause-specific mortality, and there were no differences in the incidence of major vascular events during the 5.5-year period of the trial. The GISSI prevention trial also failed to show any benefit of taking vitamin E post MI, but n-3 supplementation reduced cardiac events by 10% to 15%.[41] No CHD outcome was seen in the Heart Outcome Prevention Evaluation (HOPE) study, which also used a factorial design, in which half of patients received an antioxidant supplementation with or without ramipril.[42] In the Women's Angiographic Vitamin and Estrogen Study, postmenopausal women with coronary disease on HRT were given vitamin E and vitamin C and had unexpected significantly higher all-cause mortality rate and a trend for an increased cardiovascular mortality rate compared with the vitamin placebo women.[43] Likewise, in the HDL-Atherosclerosis Treatment Study the supplements interfered with the efficacy of statin and niacin therapy.[44]

The National Academy of Sciences of Institute of Medicine (www.iom.edu/board.asp?id=3788) has evaluated the dietary reference intake of antioxidant vitamins, selenium, and carotenoids and concluded that definite upper intake levels for those compound exist, with a lack of benefit for pharmaceutical levels of supplementation. Sources of beta-carotene and other carotenoids are yellow and orange fruits, carrots, apricots, pumpkins, green vegetables (e.g., spinach and watercress), whole milk and its products, squash, and sweet potatoes. The rich sources of vitamin E are nuts and seeds, whole grains, legumes, corn, soya, safflower, and seafood. Vitamin C is found in fruits and vegetables, citrus fruit, broccoli, green peppers, cauliflower, and brussel sprouts. Rich sources of selenium are cereals, bread, fish, liver, pork, cheese, eggs, walnuts, and Brazil nuts.

Flavonoids are polyphenols that have strong antioxidant properties. They are present in tea, apples, onions, and red wine. Generally, however, the evidence that flavonoids protect CHD is inconsistent. The cocoa beans are a rich source of flavonoid compounds. A 50-g bar of dark chocolate contains the antioxidant content of six apples, or seven onions, or two glasses of red wine.

Q: Is there any association between hyperhomocystinemia and coronary heart disease?

There is now considerable evidence from cross-sectional studies that moderate hyperhomocystinemia is associated with an increased risk of vascular events, and that elevated levels of homocysteine are an independent risk factor for both venous and arterial disease. Homocysteine is a curious sulfur-containing amino acid formed during methionine metabolism. Methionine can dimerize to homocysteine, or form disulfide bonds with proteins to produce so-called protein-bound homocysteine. In plasma about 80% of homocysteine is protein bound. Metabolism of homocysteine is by pathways that remethylate it (and which require vitamin B_{12} and folic acid), or by a transsulfuration pathway, which requires vitamin B_6. Homocysteine in blood (and elsewhere) is a product of how much methionine is eaten, mainly in protein (with about three times more methionine in animal than plant protein), and how much is metabolized (and metabolism may be affected by the amounts of B vitamins and folate available).

Causes of Hyperhomocystinemia

Plasma homocysteine can be measured by high-performance liquid chromatography or by immunoassay. Normal plasma homocysteine concentration varies between 5 and 15 μmol/L in healthy adults. Homocysteine levels above 12 μmol/L are thought to increase the CHD risk. The elevated blood levels of homocysteine can arise from different causes. The most dramatic elevations, which lead to life-threatening vascular abnormalities at a young age, are due to rare enzymatic defects at various points in the metabolic pathway (Table 6.3). A direct relation between homocysteine and cigarette smoking, diabetes, and hypertension has been suggested. An increased risk of thrombosis, associated with hyperhomocystinemia, is mediated through an interaction between

TABLE 6.3. Causes of hyperhomocystinemia

Genetic cause	Methylene tetrahydrofolate reductase (MTHER), heterozygous cystathionine synthase
Vitamin deficiency	Folic acid, vitamins B_6 and B_{12}
Systemic diseases	Hypothyroidism, liver disease, diabetic retinopathy, psoriasis, proliferative diseases (e.g., lymphoblastic leukemia)
Lifestyle factors	Physical inactivity, smoking, excessive coffee intake excessive alcohol intake
Drugs	Niacin, fibrates, antifolate agents (e.g., anticonvulsants)

inherited protein C resistance (factor V Leiden) and hyperhomocystinemia. A common polymorphism in the methylene tetrahy-
drofolate reductase (MTHFR) gene may play a role, but the effect
appears modest. Those patients who are homozygous for the
MTHFR 667 TT variant have an increased risk of only 15% to 20%
and this effect has not been observed where folate fortification is
implemented.[45,46]

Q: What does homocysteine do to arteries?
• Homocysteine generates superoxide and hydrogen peroxide,
  which damages arterial endothelium. Lowering homocysteine
  level has been shown to improve endothelial dysfunction.
• It encourages thrombosis, is proinflammatory, and accelerates
  oxidation of LDL-C.
• It prevents arterial dilatation, thus making arteries more vulnerable to obstruction.
• Homocysteine thiolactone causes platelets aggregation, and it
  interacts with LDL-C causing them to precipitate and damage
  endothelial tissue.
• It causes multiplication of arterial SMCs.

Evidence from Trials
A study showed that homocysteine levels rose inversely and monot-
onically with folate status (measured in blood or assessed in terms
of dietary intake).[47] The data of Selhub et al.[47] suggest that a large
proportion of the population, perhaps 40%, is not consuming
enough folate in the diet to keep homocysteine levels low. Folate
supplements in the range of 1 to 2 mg per day are generally
harmless, and are usually sufficient to reduce or normalize high
homocysteine levels, even if the elevation is not due to inadequate
folate consumption (<400 μg per day).

   Studies have shown the effects of homocysteine on the coagulation cascade: enhanced tissue factor activity, reduced von
Willebrand factor secretion, and inhibition of tissue plasminogen
activator binding to endothelial cells. The affinity of lipoprotein (a)
for fibrin may be increased by homocysteine concentration as low
as 8 μmol/l.[48] The Physicians' Health Study suggests that men
whose homocysteine level was above the 95th centile had 2.7 times
the risk of heart attack than those with lower levels, even after
adjusting for a variety of coronary risk factors.[49] Although early
studies reported a strong positive association between plasma
homocysteine and risk, in a recent meta-analysis, a 25% lower
homocysteine level has been associated with about a 11% lower
risk of CHD.[50] Homocysteine was measured in healthy French par-

ticipants in the Supplementation with Antioxidants and Mineral Study. The study suggested that to control homocysteine, decreasing coffee intake and increasing physical activity, dietary fiber, and folate intake might be more important in men.[51]

The Homocysteine Lowering Trialists' Collaboration reviewed data for 1114 subjects in 12 randomized trials of folic acid–based supplements to assess the effects on blood homocysteine concentrations of different doses of folic acid, with or without vitamin B_{12} and B_6, and found that reductions in blood homocysteine with folic acid supplementation were greater at higher pretreatment concentrations of homocysteine than at lower pretreatment concentration of blood folate.[52] Folic acid supplementation reduced homocysteine level by 25% and vitamin B_{12} produced an additional 7% reduction.

It should be noted that as yet most of the data on homocysteine and vascular disease are derived from cross-sectional and case-controlled studies, both of which are susceptible to bias and confounding. For instance, raised homocysteine levels are associated with declining renal function, male gender, aging, and to a variable degree with other risk factors including smoking, hypertension, raised cholesterol, and sedentary lifestyle. Data from prospective studies are inconsistent. Also, homozygosity for a defective thermolabile variant of MTHFR (a common genetic polymorphism that results in raised homocysteine) is not clearly linked with cardiovascular disease. It is therefore possible that the elevated homocysteine levels are simply a marker for established risk and of an atherogenic diet, deficient in fruit and vegetables, B vitamins, and other potentially cardioprotective nutrients. Until the results of randomized, controlled trials are available, it would be sensible to consume a diet rich in folate. Folate supplementation is not recommended as a routine preventive measure against CHD. Homocysteine measurement is useful in patients without traditional risk factors, such as renal failure or premature atherosclerosis, and helpful in differentiating high- and low-risk patients undergoing angioplasty.

Q: Do low birth weight and deprivation predispose to coronary heart disease?

People who had low birth weight or who were thin or short at birth as a result of reduced intrauterine growth have an increased rate of CHD.[53] They also have an increased prevalence of biological risk factors for the disease (e.g., hypertension, type 2 diabetes, abnormalities in lipid metabolism, and blood coagulation). Premature infants can also have an isolated reduction in insulin resistance sensitivity, which may be a risk factor for type 2 diabetes.[54] Death rates are even higher if weight "catches up" in early childhood. Death from CHD therefore may be a consequence of poor prenatal nutrition followed by improved postnatal nutrition. Unskilled men are three times more likely to die from coronary disease than professional men, according to data in a new report from the National Heart Forum. This compares with an excess mortality of only 25% in the 1970s, indicating the gap is widening.

Q: Are there any risks of exercise in ischemic heart disease sufferers?

Everyone should be encouraged to exercise, even if there is history of ischemic heart disease or previous MI, but the level of intensity would vary according to physical fitness and the severity of heart disease. Those who suffer from ischemic heart disease should exercise within the limits of angina or breathlessness and should avoid extreme cold weather and trying to walk through chest pain. There is some evidence that vigorous activity in those who have high blood pressure may increase the risk of heart attack, particularly those with other risk factors, but these patients undoubtedly benefit from moderate exercise. Inactive people should gradually increase the level of activity. Unaccustomed or infrequent physical exercise, particularly of vigorous intensity, may be hazardous in middle age.

RISK ASSESSMENT

Q: How should coronary and cardiovascular risk be assessed?

Traditionally, the risk has been assessed for CHD, but now it is advised to assess the cardiovascular risk instead. However, at present, both need to be addressed. Roughly, 20% CHD risk equals 15% CVD risk. The absolute risk should be calculated; the relative risk is for researchers only. The coronary risk is calculated as part of primary prevention, to help physicians plan treatment, such as when to prescribe lipid-lowering drugs and aspirin in the absence of established CHD. Coronary risk calculation is unnecessary in patients with established occlusive arterial disease (e.g., CHD, stroke, peripheral vascular disease, etc.) and patients with familial hyperlipidemia. Diabetes is also classified as a "coronary equivalent" for secondary prevention. Since the Framingham study is based on Caucasians, it does not reliably predict the risk for South Asians (of the Indian subcontinent), in whom it underestimates the risk. These charts also do not take family history into account. When variables such as blood pressure, cholesterol, or BMI are at their extremes, prediction is also unreliable. Predictions can be made for 1, 5, or 10 years. ATP 111 chooses 10-year CHD risk prediction, while Britain has now adopted a 10-year CVD prediction. The New Zealand charts predict CVD risk over 5 years. There is a range of charts and tables based on the Framingham data. Following are the commonly used ones:

- Sheffield table for primary prevention of CHD (3rd edition): http://bmj/contents/vol320/issue7236/large/wale3599.f1.jpeg
- New Zealand tables for absolute 5-year risk of a cardiovascular event: www.cebm.net/prognosis.asp
- Joint British Societies Coronary and Cardiovascular Risk Prediction Charts: www.bhf.org.uk/
- Framingham point scoring system (U.S. ATP 111): www.nhlbi.nih.gov/guidelines/cholesterol/risk_tbl.htm
- European SCORE Project: www.escardio.org

Joint British Societies CVD Risk Prediction Charts

The charts and the program assess the 10-year risk of CVD rather than the risk of CHD (Fig. 6.3), reflecting the treatment objective of reducing all cardiovascular events, including stroke. No chart has been provided for patients with type 2 diabetes, as they should be considered for secondary prevention. These Joint British Societies CVD risk prediction charts can also be viewed online (www.hyp.ac.uk/bhs/).

When the ratio of serum total cholesterol to LDL cholesterol exceeds 7, these charts should not be used to calculate if lipid-lowering drug needs to be prescribed. If the HDL cholesterol is not available, then assume that this is 1.00 mmol/l. High-risk people are those whose 10-year CVD risk exceeds 20% (equivalent to CHD risk of 15% over the same period). Those who have given up smoking within the past 5 years should be regarded as current smokers. These charts overestimate the risk in people under 40 years of age; therefore, clinical judgment should prevail. These charts (like all other similar charts) are based on people with untreated hypertension and untreated raised lipids. For patients who are receiving treatment, clinical judgment should be exercised. In these patients the cardiovascular risk should be assumed to be greater than that predicted by the current level of blood pressure and lipids. Cardiovascular risk is also higher than indicated in charts for patient with the following findings:

- A family history of premature CVD or stroke.
- Raised triglycerides.

Nondiabetic Men

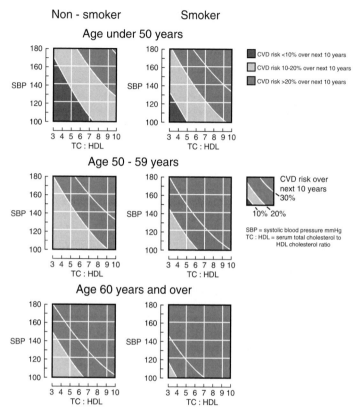

Non - smoker   Smoker

Age under 50 years

CVD risk <10% over next 10 years
CVD risk 10-20% over next 10 years
CVD risk >20% over next 10 years

Age 50 - 59 years

CVD risk over
next 10 years
30%
10% 20%

SBP = systolic blood pressure mmHg
TC : HDL = serum total cholesterol to
HDL cholesterol ratio

Age 60 years and over

FIGURE 6.3. Cardiovascular disease risk charts for nondiabetic men and women. (From the Joint British Societies. © University of Manchester.) Reproduced by kind permission of Prof Paul Durrington, University of Manchester, U.K.

- Impaired glucose tolerance.
- Asians from the Indian subcontinent, as they have 1.5 times the predicted risk.
- Target organ damage.

Framingham Scoring System Used in the United States

The Framingham scoring system is a risk assessment tool for estimating the 10-year risk of developing hard CHD (MI and coronary death).[54] The risk factors included are age, total cholesterol, HDL

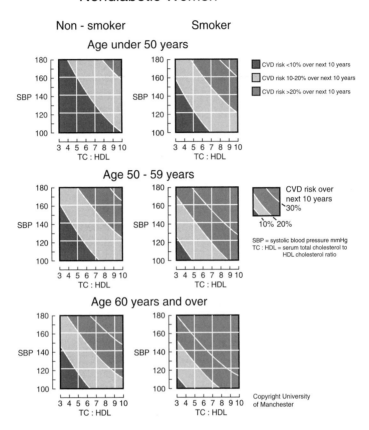

FIGURE 6.3. *Continued*

cholesterol, systolic blood pressure, treatment for hypertension, and cigarette smoking. The Framingham estimates are more accurate for total cholesterol than LDL cholesterol. Total cholesterol and HDL cholesterol should be the average of two measurements. Blood pressure readings are those at the time of assessment irrespective of treatment. Smoking means cigarette smoking during the last month. A raised HDL cholesterol level ≥60 mg/dl (>1.55 mmol/L) is considered a negative risk factor, and its presence allows for one positive risk factor to be subtracted because high HDL cholesterol levels are associated with lower CHD risk. First, calculate the number of points for each risk factor. Global risk is

TABLE 6.4. Global risk assessment / Framingham point scoring. National Institutes of Health (NIH) NHLBI publication No. 01-3305, 2001. Reproduced by kind permission of the National Heart Lung and Blood Institute, USA

Men Risk factors	Points							
	All	Age, years					Treated	
		20–39	40–49	50–59	60–69	70–79	No	Yes
Age								
20–34	–9							
35–39	–4							
40–44	0							
45–49	3							
50–54	6							
55–59	8							
60–64	10							
65–69	11							
70–74	12							
75–79	13							
Total cholesterol, mg/dL								
<160		0	0	0	0	0		
160–199		4	3	2	1	0		
200–239		7	5	3	1	0		
240–279		9	6	4	2	1		
≥280		11	8	5	3	1		
Nonsmoker		0	0	0	0	0		
Smoker		8	5	3	1	1		
HDL cholesterol, mg/dL								
≥60	–1							
50–59	0							
40–49	1							
<40	2							
Systolic blood pressure, mm Hg								
<120							0	0
120–129							0	1
130–139							1	2
140–159							1	2
≥160							2	3

cumulative and can be determined by calculating the number of Framingham points assigned to each risk factor. The 10-year risk of MI and CHD is calculated from the total points (Table 6.4).

TABLE 6.4. *Continued*

Women Risk factors	Points							
	All	Age, years					Treated	
		20–39	40–49	50–59	60–69	70–79	No	Yes
Age								
20–34	−7							
35–39	−3							
40–44	0							
45–49	3							
50–54	6							
55–59	8							
60–64	10							
65–69	12							
70–74	14							
75–79	16							
Total cholesterol, mg/dL								
<160		0	0	0	0	0		
160–199		4	3	2	1	0		
200–239		8	6	4	2	1		
240–279		11	8	5	3	2		
≥280		13	10	7	4	2		
Nonsmoker		0	0	0	0	0		
Smoker		9	7	4	2	1		
HDL cholesterol, mg/Dl								
≥60	−1							
50–59	0							
40–49	1							
<40	2							
Systolic blood pressure, mm Hg								
<120							0	0
120–129							1	3
130–139							2	4
140–159							3	5
≥160							4	6

Q: What are the noninvasive tests that can be used for CHD risk assessment?

It is suggested that noninvasive tests may be used after global risk assessment with traditional risk factors to identify the 10-year risk.[54] The following tests could be used:

Table 6.4. *Continued*

Men		Women	
Point total	10-year risk (%)	Point total	10-year risk (%)
<0	<1	<9	<1
0	1	9	1
1	1	10	1
2	1	11	1
3	1	12	1
4	1	13	2
5	2	14	2
6	2	15	3
7	3	16	4
8	4	17	5
9	5	18	6
10	6	19	8
11	8	20	11
12	10	21	14
13	12	22	17
14	16	23	22
15	20	24	27
16	25	≥25	≥30
≥17	≥30		

Exercise Treadmill Test

Due to its high false-positive rate, the treadmill test is not recommended as a screening tool. However, ischemic changes at low workload indicate an increased risk of cardiac events. ST depression of ≥1 mm within 6 minutes on the Bruce protocol indicates an increased risk of cardiovascular events in men; the absolute risk in the absence of a risk factor is low. In symptomatic patients with at least one risk factor, treadmill testing may indicate the prognosis. At present this test is indicated for men over 40 years of age with one or more risk factors in whom an intensive exercise program is recommended. Men who have one or more risk factors and show two abnormalities on treadmill testing have a 30-fold increase in 5-year cardiac risk as compared to men without a risk factor.

Electron Beam Computed Tomography (EBCT)

This is a highly sensitive technique in detecting calcium, a marker of atherosclerosis within coronary arteries, particularly in the context of multivessel disease. However, it is less sensitive than intravascular ultrasound. EBCT is not suitable for wider screening.

Magnetic Resonance Coronary Angiography (MRCA)

This test can detect only large stenosis and is capable of identifying plaque composition and size, which may locate areas that are prone to rupture. Its specificity and sensitivity are variable and not firmly established.

Positron Emission Tomography (PET)

This test can help assess blood flow through coronary arteries but has limited use because of its inability to detect coronary stenosis less than 50%. PET may have a role in the future in the detection of early endothelial function, monitoring, or aggressive lipid-lowering drug therapy and risk stratification of high-risk asymptomatic patients.

Ankle-Brachial Blood Pressure Index Testing (ABI)

ABI-detectable peripheral arterial disease has been shown to co-relate with a high prevalence of CHD. This technique is particularly useful in patients with multiple risk factors.

B-Mode Ultrasound

This test enables visualizing intima-media thickness (IMT) in the lumen of the carotid and femoral arteries. There is evidence that IMT measurements co-relate with the presence of coronary atherosclerosis and represent an independent risk factor for CHD events and stroke.

Serum Markers

The role of lipids and lipoproteins, lipoprotein (a), CRP, and homocysteine has been discussed earlier in the chapter.

PREVENTION

Q: What steps should be taken in the prevention of ischemic cardiac events?

Primary Prevention

The following essential steps are needed to prevent new-onset CHD:

- Identify a high-risk person.
- Reduce the risk factors for CHD.
- To achieve long-term benefit, all categorical risk factors should be managed.

The following practical steps are recommended:

- Risk assessment should start at the age of 20 years.
- Family history, lifestyle factors (smoking, diet, alcohol intake, physical activity, etc.) should be assessed.
- BP, BMI, and waist circumference should be recorded every 5 years, or earlier if indicated.
- Fasting lipids and blood sugar should be tested every 5 years, or if risk exists, then annually.
- Global risk assessment should be done every 5 years; if risk exists, then every 2 years.
- Provide lifestyle modification and education.
- Identify a high-risk person by calculating the CVD or CHD risk rate.
- Prevent recurrent CHD events and clinically established CHD.

After calculating the risk rate, the following steps should be taken:

People with a 10-year CHD risk <15%
Most people do not require treatment. They should be reassured and offered advice on diet and lifestyle. Their 10-year risk of CHD should be reassessed after 3 to 5 years. However, blood pressure, blood glucose, and blood lipids should be treated appropriately.

People with a 10-year CHD risk >15%
- Prescribe smoking cessation, using nicotine patches or bupropion if required.
- Attend to other modifiable factors (e.g., physical activity, diet, alcohol consumption, weight, and diabetes).
- Maintain blood pressure (<140/90, <130/80 in diabetic and renal insufficiency) and blood sugar at the target level.
- Prescribe low-dose aspirin (75–160 mg) for those in a high-risk group or those with a 10-year CHD risk ≥10%. Aspirin at 75 to 160 mg is as effective as high doses.
- Provide statin and dietary advice as discussed in Chapter 2.

Primary Prevention (British Hypertensive Society Guidelines)
Low-dose aspirin (75 mg/day) is recommended if the hypertensive patient is at least 50 years of age with BP controlled to <150/90 mm Hg and a 10-year risk of CVD of ≥20%. Statins should be used up to 80 years of age, with a 10-year risk of CVD of ≥20% and total cholesterol is lowered by 25% or LDL-C by 30% or to achieve total cholesterol <4.0 mmol/L or LDL-C <2.0 mmol/L, whichever is lower.

Aspirin irreversibly blocks the enzyme cyclooxygenase and reduces the synthesis of various prostanoids, including thromboxane A_2, a potent vasoconstrictor and platelet aggregant. Inhibition of platelet function produces an antithrombotic effect. Aspirin in primary prevention has been evaluated in the Physicians' Health Study,[55] the Hypertension Optimum Trial (HOT) Study,[56] and the Thrombosis Prevention Trial.[57] These trials reported significant reduction overall of between 32% and 44% in risk of first MI, using daily doses between 75 and 325 mg.

Secondary Prevention
The following steps be considered:

- Address lifestyle factors (e.g., smoking cessation, dietary, exercise, etc.).
- Prescribe drugs (e.g., lipid-lowering drugs, antiplatelet therapy, anticoagulants, beta-blockers, ACE inhibitors, ARBs, aldosterone, amiodarone (patients at risk of arrhythmia). Their role was discussed in earlier chapters.
- Others (e.g., cardiac rehabilitation, psychosocial treatment, stress management).

A cardiac rehabilitation program with exercise at 3-year follow-up suggested that the risk of cardiovascular mortality was reduced by 22%, a fatal second or subsequent heart attack by 25%, and total mortality by 20%.[58] A cardioprotective diet should be prescribed. No trial has been undertaken to assess the effects of weight reduction in secondary prevention, but weight reduction should become part of secondary prevention.

British Hypertensive Society

Guidelines
Aspirin should be given to all patients unless contraindicated. Statins should be prescribed in sufficient doses to all patients and lowered as in primary prevention.

Q: How do the risk factors for heart disease in women differ from those in men?
Among U.S. women, more than one half million deaths per year are attributable to CHD, more than the next seven causes of death in women combined. This figure is expected to increase in the first decade of the 21st century as the population ages. Both physicians

and women themselves underestimate the risk of heart disease in women. The Framingham data show that men with diabetes had 10-year risk of CHD of >20% in contrast to women, who rarely exceeded the 20% level.

It is well documented that women live longer than men, and this disparity is very much due to CHD. This could be a gender-mediated difference that is most simply explained by differences in sex hormones. In addition to estrogen, women have other protective factors: less central or upper body obesity, higher HDL cholesterol, and lower triglyceride levels. However, women have higher blood pressure (50% at the age of >45 years), higher levels of cholesterol (40% at the age of >55 years), higher fibrinogen levels, higher obesity rates, and a greater prevalence of diabetes than do men. Also, 25% of women report no regular sustained physical activity.[59] Low HDL levels are predictive of CHD in women and appear to be a stronger risk factor for women aged >65 years than men of similar age. Triglycerides may be a significant risk factor in women, especially older women.

Increased prevalence of obesity and diabetes in women is a contributing factor. Women have a higher frequency of angina/chest pain than men. However, women have a lower prevalence of obstructive CAD compared to men with similar symptoms. Women face worse prognosis after AMI, and older women with CAD often have greater comorbidities that influence their outcome adversely after AMI or revascularization than do men.

Women when presenting with acute coronary syndrome are also less likely to receive effective acute diagnostic and treatment strategies than men.[60] When women develop CAD, they have greater expression of their disease. It is well known that chest pain in women is less likely to be associated with flow-limiting coronary stenosis than is chest pain in men.[61] Gender differences in the endogenous pain-modulating system may contribute to differences in pain perception. The Women's Ischemic Evaluation (WISE) study suggested that chest pain without flow-limiting lesions by angiography may be associated with endothelial dysfunction and impaired coronary flow reserves.[61]

Management of heart disease in women is complicated by several factors. Perception of heart disease risk is lower among women, but the risk profile is changing as more women take up smoking. Women with CHD present later than men and have less clear-cut symptoms. Coronary heart disease presents with symptoms less frequently in women before menopause unless they have other associated risks (e.g., diabetes, family history of premature coronary disease, or raised lipids). They also present with different symptoms. They are usually 10 years older than men when they first develop symptoms and do worse than men at all ages. They present with vague chest pains, and the results of investigations can be difficult to interpret. In one in four patients, symptoms prove to be unrelated to heart disease. This may be one of the reasons why women are less likely than men to be investigated for other risk factors or to be treated with cholesterol-lowering drugs. Additionally, investigation of chest pain in women is more difficult than in men, and referral for a revascularization procedure is less common in women. There is higher prevalence of false-positive treadmill tests and exercise electrocardiograms.

Women are less likely to survive a heart attack (the first CV event is often fatal in women) or to be admitted to coronary care unit within 12 hours of a heart attack; if they do get admitted within that time scale, they are less likely to receive thrombolytic drugs. Those undergoing surgery do less well, develop more complications, and are more likely to die than men.

Other forms of atherosclerotic/thrombotic CVD, such as PAD, are critically important in women.[62] In women secondary prevention needs to be more aggressive. Lifestyle interventions are the same as in men. For weight reduction both a lifestyle and a behavioral approach should be followed.

Central Obesity
Central obesity has been shown to produce an increased risk of cardiovascular disease, particularly in women. It is possible that obesity affecting the lower part of body is not that unfavorable a factor.

Diabetes and Insulin Resistance
Diabetes is a powerful risk factor in women, increasing the CHD risk two to seven times compared with two to three times in men. Those who suffer from diabetes assume a risk of heart disease that closely approaches that of men and that is not entirely explained by the other classic heart disease risk factors. It is not understood whether the risk is independent of upper body obesity, lower HDL cholesterol levels, and higher triglyceride levels seen in women with diabetes. Raised triglycerides is a risk factor for heart disease, particularly in women. In men hyperinsulinemia increases the risk of heart disease but not in women, which could be because women possess inherent protection against insulin resistance. Diabetes patients who present with chest pain even before menopause require careful investigations. Coronary heart disease presents with symptoms less frequently in women before menopause, unless they

have other associated risks (e.g., diabetes, family history of premature coronary disease, or raised lipids).

Menopause

Studies show that around age 50 years, the female LDL level increases and still remains higher than the level seen in men. HDL levels begin to fall several years before the last menstrual period, whereas the LDL rise is much more coincidental with the cessation of menses. Menopause-related changes were greater in HDL and LDL than the lipid changes associated due to aging in the absence of menopause.

References

1. Ross R. The pathogenesis of atherosclerosis: a prospective of the 1990's. Nature 1993;362(29):801–809.
2. Stary HC, Chandler AB, et al. A definition of advanced types of atherosclerosis: a report from the Committee on Vascular Lesions of the Council on Arteriosclerosis, American Heart Association. Circulation 1995;5:1355–1374.
3. Steinberg D, Parthasarathy S, Carew T, et al. Beyond cholesterol: modification of low-density lipoprotein that increases its atherogenicity. N Engl J Med 1989;320:915–924.
4. Davies MJ. Pathology and morphology of atherosclerosis. Br J Cardiol 1997;4(suppl 1):4–10.
5. Meir J, Ridker P, Stampher M. Risk factor criterion. Circulation 2004;109(suppl IV):3–5.
6. Engstrom G, Hedblad B, Staven L. Fatality of future coronary events is related to inflammation-sensitive plasma proteins. Circulation 2004; 110:27–31.
7. Hulley S, Grady D, Bush T, et al, for the Heart and Estrogen/Progestin Replacement Study (HERS) Group. Randomised trial of estrogen plus progestin for secondary prevention of CHD in post menopausakl women. JAMA 1998;280:605–613.
8. Rossouw JE, Anderson GL, Prentice RL, et al. Writing Group for the Women's Health Initiative Investigators. Risks and benefits of estrogen plus progestin in healthy postmenopausal women: principal results from the Women's Health Initiative randomized controlled trial. JAMA 2002;288(3):321–333.
9. Giuliano F, Leriche A, Jaudinott, et al. Erectile Dysfunction in Patients with Diabetes and/or Hypertension. Rome: ESSIR, 2001.
10. Billups K, Friedrich S. Assessment of fasting lipid panels and Doppler ultrasound testing in men presenting with erectile dysfunction and no other medical problems. 95th Annual Meeting of the American Urological Association. 2002, Atlanta, GA. Abstract 655.
11. Pritzker MR. The penile stress test: a window to the heart of man? In 72nd Scientific session of the American Heart Association, 1999, Atlanta.

12. Gazzaruso C, Giordanetti S, De Amici E, et al. Relationship between ED and silent myocardial ischaemia in apparently uncomplicated diabetes 2 patients. Circulation 2004;110:22–26.

13. Hacket GI. Impotence—the most neglected complication of diabetes type 2. Diabetes Res 1995;28:75–83.

14. Klausen IC, Sjol A, Hansen PS, et al. Apolipoprotein (a) isoforms and coronary heart disease in men. A nested case-control study. Atherosclerosis 1997;132:77–84.

15. Santica M, Marlys L, Koschinsky L. Lipoprotein (a) concentration, apolipoprotein (a) size. Circulation 1999;100:1151–1154.

16. Carmena R, Duriez P, Fruchart J. Thermogenic lipoprotein particles in atherosclerosis. Circulation 2004;109(suppl 111):2–7.

17. Gullette EC, Blumenthat JA, Babyak M, et al. Effects of mental stress on left ventricular and peripheral vascular performance in patients with coronary artery disease. JAMA 1997;277:1521–1526.

18. Steptoe A. Psychosocial factors in the aetiology of coronary heart disease. Heart J 1999;82:258–259.

19. Barefoot JC, Peterson BL, Herrell FE, et al. Type A behavior and survival: a follow-up study of 1,467 patients with coronary artery disease. Am J Cardiol 1989;64:427–432.

20. Wolf PA, Kannel WB, Sorlie P, et al. Asymptomatic carotid bruit and risk of stroke: the Framingham Study. JAMA 1981;245:1442–1445.

21. Ridker P, Stampfer M. A comparison of C-reactive protein, fibrinogen, homocysteine, lipoprotein (a), and standard cholesterol screening as predictors of peripheral arterial disease. JAMA 2001;285:2481–2485.

22. Torres JL, Ridker PM. Clinical use of high-sensitivity C-reactive protein for the prediction of adverse cardiovascular events. Curr Opin Cardiol 2003;18:471–478.

23. Ridker PM, Rifai N, Rose L, et al. Comparison of CRP and LDL-C levels in the prediction of first cardiovascular events. N Engl J Med 2002;347:1557–1565.

24. Ridker PM, Brown NJ, Vaughan DE, et al. Established and emerging plasma biomarkers in the prediction of first atheromatous event. Circulation 2004;109(suppl IV):6–19.

25. du Clos TN. Functions of CRP. Ann Med 2000;32:274–278.

26. Ridker PM, Hennekens CH, Roitmann-Johnson B, et al. Plasma concentration of sICAM-1 and risks of future myocardial infarction in apparently healthy men. (US Physician's Health Study). Lancet 1998;351:88–92.

27. Wallen NH, Held C, Rehnqvist N, et al. Elevated sICAM-1 and sVCAM-1 among patients with stable angina pectoris who suffer cardiovascular death or non-fatal myocardial infarction. Eur Heart J 1999; 14:1039–1043.

28. Willerson JT, Ridker PM. Inflammation as a cardiovascular risk factor. Circulation 2004;109(suppl II):2–10.

29. Ridker PM, Cushman M, Stampher J, et al. Inflammation, aspirin, and risk of cardiovascular disease in apparently healthy man. N Engl J Med 1997;336:937–979.

30. Dichtyl W, Nilsson L, Goncalves L, et al. VLDL activates nuclear factor. KB in endothelial cells. Circulation 1999;845:1085–1094.

31. Biasucci LM, Liuzzo G, Colizzi C, et al. Clinical use of CRP for the prognostic stratification of patients with ischemic heart disease. Ital Heart J 2001;2:164–171.

32. Libby P, Ridker PM. Inflammation and atherosclerosis. Circulation 2002; 105:1135–1143.

33. Kol A, Bourcier T, Litchman AH, et al. Chlamydial and human heat shock protein 60s active human vascular endothelial, SMCs and macrophages. J Clin Invest 1999;103:571–577.

34. Gupta S, Leatham EW, Carrington D, et al. Elevated chamydia pneumoniae antibodies, cardiovascular events, and azithromycin in male survivors of myocardial infarction. Circulation 1997;96:404–407.

35. Ong G, Tomas BJ, Mansfield AO, et al. Detection and widespread distribution of *Chlamydia pneumoniae* in the vascular bed and its possible implications. J Clin Pathol 1996;49:102–106.

36. Roivainen M, Viik-Kajander M, Palosuo T, et al. Infections, inflammations and the risk of coronary disease. Circulation 2000;101:252–257.

37. Gibbons GH, Liew C, Goodarzi MO, et al. Genetic markers. Circulation 2004;109(suppl IV):47–58.

38. Stephens NG, Parsons A, Schofield PM, et al. Randomised controlled trial of vitamin E in patients with coronary disease: Cambridge Heart Antioxidant Study (CHOAS). Lancet 1996;347:781–786.

39. Rapola JM, Virtamo J, Ripatti S, et al. Randomised trial of alpha tocopherol and beta-carotene supplements on incidence of major coronary events in men with previous myocardial infarction. Lancet 1997; 349:1715–1720.

40. MRC/BHF Heart Protection Study Collaborative Group. Cholesterol-lowering therapies and antioxidant vitamin supplementation in a wide range of patients at increased risk of CHD death: early safety and efficacy experienced. Eur Heart J 1999;20:725–741.

41. GISSI-Prevenzione Investigators. Dietary supplementation with n-3 polyunsaturated fatty acids and vitamin E after myocardial infarction: results of the (GISSI-Prevenzione Trial). Lancet 1999;354:447–455.

42. Yusuf S, Sleight P, Pogue J, et al. Effects of an ACE inhibitor, ramipril, on cardiovascular events in high-risk patients. The Heart Outcome Prevention Evaluation Study Investigators (HOPE). N Engl J Med 2000;342:145.

43. Walters DD, Alderman EL, Hsia J, et al. Effects of HRT and antioxidant vitamin supplementation on coronary atherosclerosis in post-menopausal women. JAMA 2002;288:2432–2440.

44. Brown BG, Zhau XQ, Chait A, et al. Simvastatin and niacin, antioxidant vitamin or the combination for the prevention of coronary disease. N Engl J Med 2001;345:1585–1592.

45. Jacques PF, Boston AG, Wilson PW, et al. Determinants of plasma total homocysteine concentration in Framingham offspring cohort. Am J Clin Nutri 2001;73:613–621.

46. Klerk M, Verhoef P, Clarke R, et al. MTHFR 667C→ T polymorphism and risk of CHD: a meta-analysis. JAMA 2002;288:2023–2031.

47. Selhub J, Jacques PF, Wilson PWF, et al. Vitamin status and intake as primary determinants of homocysteinemia in an elderly population. JAMA 1993;270(22):2726–2727.

48. Refsum H, Ueland PM, Nygard O, et al. Homocysteine and cardiovascular disease. Annu Rev Med 1998;49:31–62.

49. Stamfer MJ, Malinow MR, Willer MC, et al. Physicians' Health Study. A prospective study of plasma homocysteine and risk of myocardial infarction in US physicians. JAMA 1992;268:877–879.

50. Wald DS, Law M, Morris JK, et al. Homocystine and cardiovascular disease. BMJ 2002;325:1202.

51. Mennen LI, de Courcy GP, Guilland JC, et al. Homocysteine, cardiovascular factors, and habitual diet in the French supplementation with antioxidant vitamin and mineral study. Am J Clin Nutr 2002;76: 1279–1289.

52. Homocysteine Trialists' Collaboration. Lowering blood homocysteine with folic acid based supplements: meta-analysis of randomised trials. BMJ 1998;316:894–898.

53. Martyn CN, Barker DJP, Osmond C. Mother's pelvic size, foetal growth, death from stroke and CHD in men in UK. Lancet 1996;348:1264–1268.

54. Grundy SM, Balady GJ, Criqui M, et al. Primary prevention of CHD guidance from Framingham statement for health care professionals from American Heart Association's task force on risk reduction. Circulation 1998;97:1876–1887.

55. The streering committee of the Physician's Health Study Research group. Final report on the aspirin component of the ongoing Physicians' Health Study. N Engl J Med 1989;321:129–135.

56. Medical Research Council's general practice research framework. Thrombosis prevention trial. Lancet 1998;351:233–241.

57. Collaborative Group of the Primary Prevention Project. Low-dose aspirin and vitamin E in people at cardiovascular risk. Lancet 2001; 357:89–95.

58. O'Conner GT, Buring JE, Yusuf S, et al. An overview of randomised trials of rehabilitation with exercise after myocardial infarction. Circulation 1989;80:234–244.

59. Mosca L, Grundy MD, Scott M, et al. AHA/ACC scientific statement. Guide to preventive cardiology for women. Circulation 1999;99: 2080–2084.

60. Maynard C, Beshansky JR, Griffith JL, et al. Influence of sex on the use of cardiac procedures in patients presenting to the emergency department. Circulation 1996;94(suppl 9):93–98.

61. Merz CN, Kelsey S, Pepine CJ, et al. The Women's Ischemic Evaluation (WISE) study. J Am Coll Cardol 1999;33:1453–1461.

62. AHA Statement. Evidence based guidelines for cardiovascular prevention in women. Circulation 2004;109:672–693.

Chapter 7
Chronic Stable Angina

The annual incidence of angina pectoris in the United Kingdom is 0.5%; the male to female ratio is 2 : 1. More than 1.4 million people suffer from angina, and 300,000 have a heart attack every year.

DIAGNOSIS

Q: How does atypical angina differ from typical angina?

Angina pectoris is a clinical syndrome characterized by discomfort in the chest, jaw, shoulder, back, or arms. It is typically aggravated by exercise or emotional stress and relieved by nitroglycerin. Anginal pain occurs when at least one coronary artery (obstructive coronary artery disease [CAD]) is involved, but can also present in patients with valvular heart disease, hypertrophic cardiomyopathy, and uncontrolled hypertension. Although the term *angina* usually refers to chronic stable type, there are three types: chronic stable angina, atypical angina, and unstable angina. Unstable angina is now classified as an acute coronary syndrome (ACS).

Anginal symptoms are initially experienced on exertion, which is termed angina of effort. Most symptomatic patients have the lumen of one or more segments of their artery reduced by at least half. Over half the patients show recanalization through the thrombus. There are many variations in the size and shape of the thrombus. Angina can be classified according to the severity of the symptoms (Table 7.1).

Chest pain is the most common mode of presentation. The pain lasts for no more than 10 to 15 minutes. The character of pain may be of crushing, compressing, stabbing, choking, or burning type. The site of pain is usually retrosternal, spreading to both sides of the anterior chest but most commonly to the left. The pain classically radiates along the inner aspect of the left upper limb but may do so to the neck, shoulder, and jaw. Tingling along the left upper limb or fingers may be felt. Breathlessness may accompany pain or may be the only symptom. Fatigue and perspiration may coexist.

TABLE 7.1. Grading of angina by the Canadian Cardiovascular Society and the New York Heart Association.[1]

Class	Canadian Cardiovascular Society*	New York Heart Association
I	Angina occurs with strenuous exercise	Patient has cardiac disease, no symptoms
II	Angina occurs on climbing stairs rapidly	Patient has cardiac disease, no symptoms at rest but occur on ordinary activities
III	Angina occurs on climbing one flight of stairs	Patient has cardiac disease, no symptoms at rest but occur on less ordinary activities
IV	Symptoms present at rest, inability to do ordinary activity comfortably	Patient has cardiac disease, symptom at rest, inability to perform significant activity

*From Campeau.[17]

The predisposing factors include eating a heavy meal, cold weather, stress, and sexual intercourse. Stress may be in the form of anger, fright, anxiety, or arguments. Coronary spasm may occur both in normal and diseased vessels, which may precipitate anginal symptoms. The symptoms depend on the severity of the spasm. The cause of coronary spasm is not clear. It is possible that certain sites in the coronary artery are more prone to spasm. Since an atheromatous lesion has acquired hypersensitivity to vasoconstrictors, one possibility is that the endothelium at this site is deficient in the production of endothelial-derived relaxant factor. Endothelial damage itself increases sensitivity to vasoconstrictor stimuli. Anginal pain should be distinguished from other causes of chest pain, such as anxiety and hyperacidity, and from pain of musculoskeletal origin. The physical examination is usually unremarkable. However, during an anginal attack increased blood pressure and increase heart rate may be noticed due to an augmented sympathetic response. Mitral regurgitation due to muscle dysfunction may be detected.

Atypical angina (vasospastic, Prinzmetal's angina) is a rare form of angina and is more commonly prevalent in women. Prinzmetal first described it. Unlike stable angina, coronary spasm has no relation with exercise but is the cause of myocardial ischemia. On the contrary, the pain is sometimes relieved with exercise. The pain usually comes while resting or sleeping. The electrocardiogram may show ST elevation. The pain is relieved by glycerine trinitrate. Specialist investigations using provocative tests (e.g., hyperventilation, cold-pressor testing, or ergometrine challenge) may be required to make the diagnosis. Ventricular arrhythmia and heart block may occur. Calcium channel blockers (CCBs) may prevent coronary spasm, but beta-blockers may worsen the symptoms. However, patients may remain symptom-free for months or years. Like unstable angina, there is a subsequent risk of heart attack.

Q: Who should be referred for investigations for angina?

Referral is required for the following situations:

- All newly diagnosed cases of angina, for an objective assessment of myocardial ischemia.
- For diagnostic or prognostic reasons or where a positive diagnosis would have major implications for the patient's livelihood.
- For treatment for patients of any age with severe, unstable, or rapidly progressive symptoms, for patients with secondary angina from remediable cause, or for patients with unacceptable symptoms despite adequate medical treatment.

Urgent referral, depending on the severity of symptoms, is required for the following situations:

- Patients with recent-onset angina or stable angina but with severe symptoms, or with a previous history of heart attack or heart failure.
- Patients who suffer angina pain at rest, a sudden increase in severity or frequency of angina, or recent onset of angina not responding to medical treatment.

Q: What investigations are advocated for a patient suspected of having angina?

Clinical history and examination are very important. The speed with which the investigations are undertaken depends on the urgency, taking into account the age of the patient, the presence of other risk factors, the severity of chest pain, the likelihood of the diagnosis, and the findings on clinical examination. Chest x-ray helps to exclude congestive heart failure, valvular lesions, pericardial disease, or aortic dissection/aneurysm. However, the use of routine chest x-ray is not well established.

Blood tests should include tests for anemia, thyroid function, urea, electrolytes, lipid profile, glucose and cardiac enzymes, troponin, erythrocyte sedimentation rate (ESR) and high-sensitivity C-reactive protein (hsCRP). Resting electrocardiogram (ECG) is indicated in all cases as an initial test, although a normal ECG does not exclude CAD. Evidence of a prior Q-wave on ECG and evidence of left ventricular hypertrophy also increases the probability of angina. If the resting ECG is normal, depending on the likelihood of the diagnosis, treadmill stress testing is arranged. The treadmill test is most valuable when the pretest probability is intermediate, for example, when a 50-year-old man has atypical angina and the probability of CAD is about 50%.[2] When the probability of CAD is high, a positive test result only confirms the high probability of disease, and a negative test result may not decrease the probability of CAD enough to make a clinical difference. When the probability of CAD is very low, a negative test result only confirms the low probability of disease; a positive test may not increase the probability of disease enough to make a clinical difference.[2] If there is high suspicion of CAD, then exercise testing could be combined with thallium testing (myocardial perfusion imaging [MPI]) or angiography.

Echocardiography is usually not indicated in most patients, unless valvular disease or hypertrophic cardiomyopathy is suspected. Coronary angiography is very important in the diagnosis where myocardial ischemia is suspected and noninvasive testing is contraindicated. The recommendations are for cardiac stress imaging as the initial test in the following situations[2]:

1. Exercise ECG for the diagnosis of obstructive CAD
2. Exercise myocardial perfusion imaging or exercise echocardiography when the patient has intermediate pretest probability of CAD or has either Wolff-Parkinson-White syndrome or more than 1 mm of rest ST depression
3. Exercise MPI or exercise echocardiography if there is a past history of revascularization
4. If a patient is not able to exercise, then adenosine or dipyridamol MPI or dobutamine echocardiography is indicated if patient has either an intermediate pretest probability of CAD or a past history of revascularization.

When the probability of severe angina is low, noninvasive tests are most appropriate. However, when the pretest probability is high, direct referral for coronary angiography is a suitable choice. Coronary angiography is most useful in the following situations (also, see Chapter 5):

1. If a patient suspected of CAD survived sudden cardiac death
2. Uncertain diagnosis after noninvasive tests

3. If the patient is unable to undergo noninvasive tests.
4. Patients in whom coronary artery spasm is suspected and provocative tests may be necessary.
5. Patients with a pretest probability of left main stem or three-vessel disease.
6. Occupational requirement for a firm diagnosis.
7. To exclude anatomical anomalies in young patients as the cause of angina.

PROGNOSIS AND TREATMENT

Q: What are the tests for risk assessment and prognosis in a patient with chronic stable angina?
The following factors are associated with worse prognosis:

- One of the strongest and most consistent prognostic markers is the maximum exercise capacity. Poor exercise tolerance, either due to myocardial ischemia or left ventricular dysfunction, is a bad marker.
- Another important prognostic marker is related to exercise-induced ischemia. ST-segment depression and elevation (in leads without pathological Q waves and not in aVR) best summarize the prognostic information related to ischemia.[2]
- Left ventricular dysfunction or ejection fraction is less than 40%.
- Exercise stress test shows ST segment depression >2 mm, poor exercise tolerance, or a fall of blood pressure.
- Myocardial perfusion test shows thallium uptake in the lungs.
- Angiography shows left main-stem involvement or multivessel disease, especially in the presence of left ventricular systolic dysfunction.
- Chest x-ray shows cardiomegaly, left ventricular aneurysm, or pulmonary venous congestion.
- A family history of myocardial infarction (MI) and diabetes is an independent predictor of death for coronary heart disease (CHD).
- Increasing age.
- Male gender, but after menopause females have a similar risk.

Stress imaging tests such as the radionuclide MPI test or two-dimensional echocardiography at rest and during stress are valuable for the purpose of risk stratification and planning the best route of management. A normal thallium scan is highly indicative of a benign prognosis even in patients with known CHD. Coronary angiography is usually not indicated unless other measures show high risk. Stress echocardiography is also able to provide additional prognostic information.

Q: What are the drugs of choice for the treatment of angina?

The aim of treatment is to decrease the frequency of anginal attack, control symptoms, prevent MI, and prolong survival. Treatment of angina can be considered under the following headings:

- Managing risk factors (e.g., smoking cessation; treating hypertension, diabetes and elevated LDL-C; weight reduction in all obese patients, and consuming a Mediterranean-type/cardioprotective/TLC diet).
- Relief of symptoms with medical treatment.
- Coronary revascularization.
- Rehabilitation.

In stable angina, aspirin (75 mg daily) reduces the risk of acute MI (AMI) and sudden death by 34%.[3] Similarly, 325 mg aspirin reduces mortality and morbidity by 20% in the International Study of Infarct Survival (ISIS-2).[4] If a patient is allergic to aspirin, clopidogrel is an alternative.[5]

Four groups of drugs are used in the prevention and treatment of angina: nitrates, beta-blockers, CCBs, and potassium channel activators. Nitrates, CCBs, and potassium channel activators are vasodilators. There is no direct evidence that any of these agents has a significant effect on the incidence of sudden death or heart attack. There is little evidence for the intrinsic superiority of one group of drugs over another in terms of symptom relief. It is, however, possible that the combination of two antianginal drugs is more efficient than using one. There is also the added advantage of reduced side effects. Precaution should be taken when discontinuing these drugs. They should be slowly tapered off unless serious side effects are experienced. Rapid-acting nitrates relieve acute angina and may also be used prophylactically in situations likely to induce an attack. Beta-blockers and long-acting nitrates can be used for long-term management of chronic stabile angina.

NITRATES

Glycerine trinitrate (GTN) is a short-acting drug, whereas glycerine mononitrate and glycerine dinitrate are longer-acting. Nitrates cause coronary dilatation, which improves myocardial circulation, and venodilatation, which reduces venous return to the heart, thus reducing the cardiac workload. The latter is the predominant effect. Nitrates thus reduce myocardial ischemia, relieve pain, and improve exercise tolerance. In patients with exertional stable angina, long-acting nitrates improve exercise tolerance, increase the time to onset of angina, and decrease ST-segment depression during exercise tolerance. However, there is no evidence that they reduce mortality in a patient with chronic stable angina. Headache is the most troublesome symptom. Hypotension, especially postural hypotension, may occur. This tends to become less frequent after a few days. Nitrates are available as sublingual tablets or spray, oral modified-release preparations, transdermal patches, or 2% ointment of glycerine trinitrate for topical use. Skin reactions can occur with local applications, caused by the drug or its vehicle.

Glycerine trinitrate taken as sublingual tablets in the dose of 300 or 500 μg, or sublingual spray in the dose of 0.3 to 1.0 mg relieves chest pain in 10 seconds, and the effect lasts for 20–30 minutes. Oral tablets lose effective in 12 weeks; therefore, if they these are used infrequently, sublingual spray is preferred. Isosorbide dinitrate can also be taken sublingually as a 5 mg tablet or 1.25 mg spray, the effect lasting up to 1 hour. Sustained-release preparations of isosorbide mononitrate and dinitrate can be taken once a day. Isosorbide mononitrate is used in the initial dose of 20 mg two or three times a day, or 40 mg twice a day (10 mg twice a day for those who have not received nitrates previously), typically 120 mg/d for extended-release preparations. Isosorbide dinitrate is used in the dose of 5 to 20 mg sublingually, and 30 to 120 mg orally, in divided doses; maintenance dose 40 or 80 mg, 8–12 hours. If nitrates fail to control symptoms, an alternative antianginal drug should be used.

BETA-BLOCKERS

A randomized controlled trial in chronic stable angina has shown that treatment with beta-blockers is efficacious in reducing symptoms of angina and episodes of ischemia, and improving exercise capacity.[6] Beta-blockers are the drug of choice in angina and they may be used alone or in combination with nitrates. The long-term trials show that there is 23% reduction in the odds of death among MI survivors randomized to beta-blockers.[7] All beta-blockers are equally effective in angina. The heart rate should be reduced to 55 to 60 beats per minute. In more severe cases, however, heart rate should be reduced to 50 per minute, provided there are no symptoms arising from bradycardia, and heart block does not occur. Beta-blockers restrict the heart rate during exercise. Patients with angina should not increase heart rate above 100 per minute during exercise. Metoprolol, atenolol, and propranolol are quite effective in symptomatic relief. Carvedilol, bisoprolol, and metoprolol slow-release are as effective and may also be better tolerated in patients with peripheral vascular disease (PVD) and those with left ventricular dysfunction. These drugs are described in Chapter 4.

CALCIUM-CHANNEL BLOCKERS (CCBs)

Dihydropryridines (e.g., nifedipine and amlodipine), which are potent vasodilators, relieve myocardial ischemia by venodilatation (reduces myocardial demand), arterial vasodilatation (reduces resistance against the left ventricular contraction), and coronary dilatation (increases myocardial oxygen supply). Nondihydropyridines (e.g., diltiazem, verapamil) are also vasodilators, though not as potent, but they also exert their effect by depressing the myocardium, thus reducing myocardial demand. Nondihydropyridines are preferred over dihydropyridines in the absence of heart failure, as a second-line agent when there are contraindications to the use of beta-blockers, or if the patient is intolerant. They also have modest prognostic benefits. Short-acting CCBs are associated with increased incidence of MI and mortality; therefore, long-acting preparations (including slow-release) should be used. Verapamil should be avoided in Wolff-Parkinson-White syndrome and left ventricular dysfunction. Verapamil reduces cardiac events and angina post-MI.[8] Diltiazem is used as 60–120 mg tid; slow-release 90–180 mg bid. Verapamil is used as 80 mg tid, increasing to 120 mg tid.

POTASSIUM-CHANNEL ACTIVATORS

Nicorandil is the first potassium-channel activator indicated for angina. Potassium (K^+) channels conduct ions in and out of the cell and act like switches regulating cellular excitability. Nicorandil lowers arterial resistance and reduces cardiac afterload by opening K^+ channels. It also dilates venous capacitance vessels and reduces cardiac preload. In patients with coronary artery disease, it dilates both stenotic and nonstenotic coronary arteries and improves coronary blood flow. It may also prevent coronary spasm. Unlike nitrates, tolerance is not a problem.

Nicorandil is licensed in the U.K. for the prevention and long-term treatment of angina. It is used in the dose of 10 to 20 mg twice a day with maximum of 30 mg twice a day. It is effective as monotherapy but can be used with other agents. It is not proven whether it affects the risk of death or heart attack in patients with coronary artery disease. Nicorandil should not be used in patients with left ventricular failure with low filling pressure. Sildenafil and oral hypoglycemic agents (e.g., glibenclamide) interacts with nicorandil and should not be co-prescribed.

Class I (i.e., American College of Cardiology (ACC)/American Heart Association [AHA] class I measures show evidence, or there is general agreement, that a given procedure or treatment is useful and effective)[2,9]:

- Aspirin and lipid-lowering drugs reduce MI and death in anginal patient.
- Beta-blockers as initial therapy, whether or not the patient previously suffered MI, though for the former the evidence is stronger. Beta-blockers reduce mortality post-MI. However, their use in other cases is based on their capacity to reduce mortality in hypertension.
- CCBs and/or long-acting nitrates as initial therapy when beta-blockers are contraindicated, not successful, or the patient suffered side effects.
- CCBs and/or long-acting nitrates in combination with beta-blockers when initial therapy with beta-blocker is not successful.
- Sublingual nitroglycerin for immediate relief for symptoms.
- Lipid-lowering therapy in patients with proven or suspected CAD and LDL-C >130 mg/dL (3.4 mmol/L) with a target LDL-C of <100 mg/dL (2.6 mmol/L).
- Angiotensin-converting enzyme (ACE) inhibitors in patients with CAD, who has diabetes and/or LVSD.

Class IIa (ACC/AHA class IIa measures show evidence or opinion in favor of usefulness/efficacy)[2,9]:

- Clopidogrel when aspirin is contraindicated.
- Long-acting nondihydropyridine CCBs instead of beta-blockers as initial therapy.
- Lipid-lowering therapy in patients with proved or suspected CAD (see Chapter 2).
- ACE inhibitors in all patients with significant CAD or other vascular disease.
- Surgical laser transmyocardial revascularization (TMR) as an alternative therapy for chronic stable angina in patients refractory to medical therapy who are not candidates for percutaneous interventions or revascularization.

Q: How should one proceed with the choice of antianginal drugs?
- First step: glyerine trinitrate.
- Second step: add beta-blocker especially if previous history of MI; if contraindicated, add CCBs.
- Third step: add CCBs; if contraindicated, add long-acting nitrate.

If a patient suffers pain at rest and nocturnal pain, suggesting vasospasm, initiate therapy with long-acting nitrates and CCBs. All patients should have sublingual spray for prophylaxis before exercise and for symptomatic relief of symptoms. A cardioselective beta-blocker is the first choice, except in patients with ventricular arrhythmia, for whom sotalol is preferred. For thyrotoxic patients propranolol may be the drug of choice. In patients for whom a beta-blocker is contraindicated and in those who suffer from coronary artery spasm, hypertension, diabetes, PVD, asthma, or Raynaud's phenomenon, CCBs should be tried. Diltiazem and verapamil are equally effective. Compliance with amlodipine is better. Nifedipine, amlodipine, and felodipine are all effective. If a patient is unable to take beta-blockers and CCBs, then long-acting nitrates should be considered. If one drug is ineffective, another drug should be substituted; if necessary, combination therapy should be used. Triple therapy is of doubtful benefit. Nevertheless, at least two and preferably all three classes of drugs should be tried before giving up on medical treatment. Combined with beta-blockers or CCBs, nitrates produce greater antianginal and antiischemic effects in patients with stable angina. Use of ACE inhibitors and lipid-lowering drugs should be considered.

Q: What are the indications of angioplasty?

Percutaneous transluminal coronary angioplasty (PTCA) was originally introduced as a balloon angioplasty, a procedure that involved using a catheter-borne balloon that was inflated at the site of coronary stenosis. The scope of this procedure has widened to include the use of stents, atherectomy and laser therapy. The following are the important indications for angioplasty:

- Stable angina in patients with suitable coronary anatomy who are uncontrolled on or intolerant of medical treatment.
- Two- or three-vessel disease with significant proximal left anterior descending artery disease, in patients who have normal anatomy suitable for catheter-based therapy, normal left ventricular function, and who do not have treated diabetes.
- Unstable angina not responding to medical treatment.
- Unstable angina or AMI followed by a positive exercise test.
- AMI complicated by cardiogenic shock.
- AMI where thrombolytic drugs are contraindicated.
- One- or two-vessel disease without a significant disease of proximal left anterior descending artery but with a large area of viable myocardium and high-risk criteria on noninvasive testing.

Disadvantages

Angioplasty has similar mortality to coronary artery bypass grafting (CABG), with 1% mortality for the treatment of single-vessel disease, and 2% when more than one vessel is dilated. About 3% of people need an emergency heart bypass due to damage to the coronary artery during angioplasty. Almost one third of patients experience restenosis within 3 months and again require angioplasty. Of those who have angioplasty on more than one vessel, almost half have restenosis of one or more vessels. Almost one fifth of patients who have angioplasty require heart bypass within 3 years.

STENTS

A coronary stent (scaffold) is an artificial support device in the coronary artery to keep the vessel open. It was developed to overcome the two primary limitations of balloon angioplasty: sudden closure of the coronary artery and late restenosis. Stents prevent narrowing of the coronary artery by providing a scaffolding lattice to tack back the inner surface of the coronary artery. It prevents late restenosis by mechanically enforced remodeling and resetting of the vessel size of the stented segment. In 20% to 40%, restenosis gradually occurs.

There are several different coronary stents available, and the scaffolding lattice of each stent differs markedly in configuration. Coronary artery stenting is currently applicable only to relatively large arteries (>3 mm diameter). The stents can be categorized into the mesh stents, characterized by strong and extensive scaffolding of the vessel wall (Wallstent, Palmaz-Schatz, and AVE Micro) and the coil stents, characterized by a low metallic surface area and predominantly transverse strut orientation (Gianturco-Roubin, Wiktor, Multilink, and Cordis). Drug-eluting stents (DESs) are now used and have been shown to dramatically reduce the risk of restenosis compared with bare metal stents. In the Sirolimus-Eluting Coronary Stent (SIRUS) Trial, 1058 patients undergoing elective coronary stent implantation were randomized to a bare stent or the sirolimus DES.[10] The patients were followed-up for a year. The sirolimus stent reduced the restenosis rate by 75%, from 36.3% to 8.9%, and reduced the rate of repeat revascularization from 28.4% to 13%. No significant advantage was found with regard to mortality and MI.

Coronary stenting usually follows balloon angioplasty, which requires inserting a guide catheter at the ostium of the coronary artery through the femoral artery. The guide wire is then manipulated beyond the lesion, after which the balloon catheter is inserted over it. When this catheter is positioned at the site of blockage, it is slowly inflated to widen the coronary artery and is then removed. The stent-mounted catheter is then threaded into the artery. When this is correctly positioned in the coronary artery, the balloon is inflated, expanding the stent against the wall of coronary artery. The balloon catheter, guide wire, and guide catheter are then removed, leaving the stent. A cardiac angiography follows to ensure that the stent is keeping the artery open. Aspirin is taken for few days before the procedure in the dose of 300 mg a day. There is a small risk that the stented artery may close. Thrombosis, bleeding, and artery damage are rare complications.

Q: Do revascularization procedures have a better outcome than medical treatment?

There is no significant advantage of PTCA over medical treatment. The Randomized Intervention Treatment of Angina (RITA-2) trial compared the effectiveness of angioplasty with medical treatment in patients with one-vessel or two-vessel disease or mild to moderate angina, deemed suitable for either treatment.[11] More patients who received angioplasty died or had an MI than did patients who received medical treatment. Angioplasty also led to a greater rate of nonfatal heart attack. No difference existed between the groups for mortality, 19% of patients who received angioplasty or heart bypass compared with 23% who received medical treatment. At 3 months, angina and exercise tolerance were more improved in the angioplasty group, an effect that attenuated in 1 or 2 years. A study of one-vessel disease and mild angina also has shown that medical treatment is only slightly less efficacious in relieving symptoms and improving exercise tolerance than angioplasty, while the prognosis was comparable in both groups.[12]

In another randomized trial the outcomes of medical treatment, angioplasty, and heart bypass were compared in a patient with stable angina.[13] Mortality and MI rates do not differ for medical therapy and angioplasty in low-risk patients with single-vessel disease. In high-risk patients with multivessel disease, mortality is lower at 5, 7 and 10 years in patients who receive bypass surgery rather than medical therapy. Angioplasty and bypass surgery produce similar reduced rates of mortality and MI, but the need for repeat revascularization is more common after angioplasty. In the presence of heart failure, medical treatment with ACE inhibitors, beta-blockers, and spironolactone is probably superior for most patients.

These studies suggest that medical treatment should initially be given in cases of mild chronic angina. If this fails, revascularization should be considered. (Primary coronary angioplasty is described in Chapter 8.)

Q: What are the indications for coronary artery bypass grafting?
Coronary artery bypass grafting (CABG) is now an established success; some 25,000 operations are performed each year in the U.K., with an operative mortality now approaching 1% in most centers. New minimally invasive operative procedures that do not require cardiopulmonary bypass may extend its use to patients who are at greater risk of surgery. Arterial grafts can be used not only from the internal mammary artery but also from the right gastroepiploic artery, inferior epigastric artery, and radial artery. Arterial grafts have many advantages over saphenous vein grafts. They have a reduced propensity to develop atherosclerosis. Reviews of patients treated with internal mammary artery grafting of left anterior descending artery have shown improved long-term survival, a lower long-term incidence of angina, and higher graft patency rates. Fourteen percent of coronary bypass operations are now reoperations. Repeat grafting is associated with higher operative risk (3%). Symptom-free patients, without complication, can be expected to return to work in 4 to 8 weeks.

The important indications for CABG are as follows:

- Patients with significant left main artery disease.
- One- or two-vessel disease without significant proximal left anterior descending artery disease but with a large area of viable myocardium and high-risk criteria on noninvasive testing.
- Patients with three-vessel disease; the surgical benefit is better with left ventricular dysfunction (ejection <50%).
- Patients with two-vessel disease with significant proximal left anterior descending artery disease and left ventricular dysfunction (ejection <50%).
- Patients with one- or two-vessel artery disease without proximal left anterior descending artery disease who survived sudden cardiac death or sustained ventricular tachycardia.
- Patients who have not been successfully treated by medical therapy.

Q: How do the results of CABG compare with those of angioplasty?
Some patients are suitable for either procedure (CABG or PCTA). Overall there is no evidence of a major difference between the two over 3 to 5 years in the risk of death or heart attack. Occasionally, it is difficult to dilate all stenosed segments of the coronary artery at a single attempt of angioplasty, and restenosis occurs within 6 months in about one third of patients. Therefore, patients initially treated with angioplasty needed more repeat procedures to restore blood circulation (30–50%) than did bypass patients (5–10%).

Both procedures relieve angina in most patients, but overall bypass was slightly more effective at least for the first few years. Thus in the RITA-1 trial, 11% of the CABG group compared with 32% of the angioplasty group had angina 6 months after the procedure; after 2 years the comparable figures were 21% and 32%.[14] Patients undergoing angioplasty required more medications. However, with regard to physical activity, exercise tolerance, employment status, and quality of life, there was no significant difference. The two United States trials of PTCA versus CABG groups have shown that early and late survival rates have been equivalent for both groups.[15,16] In the Bypass Angioplasty Revascularization Investigation (BARI) Trial, the subgroup of patients with treated diabetes (with multiple severe lesions) had significantly better survival rates with CABG. In the Emory Angioplasty versus Surgery Trial (EAST), diabetics had equivalent survival rates with both procedures.

Patients who wish to avoid major operation can choose angioplasty provided they understand the higher risk of recurrent angina, with a one in three risk of additional procedures during the next few years. Those who prefer a more certain medium-term result may choose bypass, but with no greater overall risk of mortality or major morbidity. Patients with single-vessel disease also do not have a prognostic benefit with CABG.

Q: What are the newer revascular techniques and their advantages?
The following are some of the newer techniques:

Coronary Atherectomy Devices
Since PTCA does not remove the plaque but acts by splitting and shifting the plaque and stretching the coronary artery, this led to the development of new devices that remove the plaque and also cause fewer traumas to the deeper components of the arterial wall. Atherectomy devices include directional, rotational atherectomy, transluminal extraction, and excimer laser angioplasty.

The directional coronary atherectomy is a nonballoon interventional device. It is a cutting device, as it cuts the plaque and leaves smooth lumen. It is a suitable procedure when lesions are ostial, eccentric, or present at bifurcations. Its contraindications include small vessel size, calcified lesions, lesion angulation, and proximal tortuosity of the vessel.

Rotational atherectomy ablates plaque material. Percutaneous rotational atherectomy uses a high-speed metal burr coated with diamond clips to abrade and destroy plaques into fine microparticles. This technique is suitable for harder calcified, fibrotic lesions.

It is contraindicated in patients with left ventricular dysfunction and in those with visible thrombus.

Transluminal extraction atherectomy (TEC) increases luminal size by cutting material and aspirating it. The system comprises a conical cutting head with two stainless steel blades bound to the distal end of a hollow flexible torque tube. A suction bottle, which collects the excised lesions, and a battery-powered motor drive unit are attached to the proximal end of the tube. The TEC is useful in lesions in which thrombus or debris has to be removed from the artery.

Coronary Laser Angioplasty

Coronary laser angioplasty involves using excimer laser systems. It is a pulsed laser, that is, the energy is released in short bursts of ultraviolet light separated by relatively long periods of silence, during which laser emission is switched off. This procedure is indicated in saphenous vein graft lesions, long lesions, osteal lesions, and total occlusions. Its contraindications include bifurcation lesions, highly eccentric lesions, severe lesion, angulation, vessel tortuosity, and prior dissection.

Transmyocardial Laser Revascularization (TMR)

Transmyocardial laser revascularization with the aid of a laser makes small channels into the myocardium, which lead to improved exercise tolerance. The Atlantic Study showed that TMR improved exercise tolerance in intractable angina on maximum medical treatment.[17] The procedure is performed in the operating theater (with carbon dioxide or holmium: yttrium-aluminum-garnet [YAG] laser) or by a percutaneous approach. Although this technique gives symptomatic improvement in chronic stable angina, no definite benefits have been shown in terms of increasing myocardium perfusion.

Spinal Cord Stimulation

This method involves accurate placement of the stimulating electrode in the dorsal epidural space, usually at the C7-T1 level. This method is proposed for patients with chronic stable angina refractory to medical, catheter intervention, and surgical therapy.

References

1. Campeau L. Grading of angina pectoris (Letter). Circulation 1976; 54(3):522–523.
2. Gibbons RJ, Chatterjee K, Daley J, et al. ACC/AHA/ACP guidelines for the management of patients with chronic stable angina. Circulation 1999;99:2829–2848.

3. Juul-Mollers, Edvardson N, Jahumatz B, et al., for Swedish Angina Pectoris Aspirin Trial (SAPAT) group. Double blind trial of aspirin in primary prevention of MI in patients with stable angina. Lancet 1992;340:1421–1425.

4. ISIS-2 Collaborators. International Study of Infarct Survival 2. Lancet 1998;2:349–360.

5. CAPRI Steering Committee. A randomised, blinded trial of clopidogrel vs. aspirin in patients at risk of ischaemic events. Lancet 1996;348: 1329–1339.

6. Dargie HJ, Ford I, Fox KM. Total Ischemic Burden European Trial (TIBET). Effects of ischemia and treatment with atenolol, nifedipine SR and their combination on outcome in patients with chronic stable angina. Eur Heart J 1996;17:104–112.

7. Freemantle N, Cleland J, Young P, et al. Beta blockade after myocardial infarction: systemic review and meta regression analysis. BMJ 1999;318:1730–1737.

8. DAVITT Group. The Danish Verapamil Infarction Trial. Am J Cardiol 1990;66:779–785.

9. Gibbons RJ, Chatterjee K, Daley J, et al. ACC/AHA/ACP guidelines for the management of patients with chronic stable angina. Circulation 2003;107:149.

10. Cohen DJ, Bakhai A, Chunxue S, et al. Cost effectiveness of sirolimus-eluting stents for the treatment of complex coronary stenoses (SIRUS) trial. Circulation 2004;110:508–514.

11. RITA-2 Trial Participants. Coronary angioplasty vs. medical therapy for angina: the second Randomized Intervention Treatment of Angina (RITA-2). Lancet 1997;350:461–468.

12. Parsi AF, Folland ED, Hartigan P, et al. A comparison of angioplasty with medical therapy in the treatment of single-vessel coronary artery disease. N Engl J Med 1992;346:1773–1780.

13. Solomon AJ, Gersh BJ. Management of chronic stable angina; medical therapy, PTCA and CAGB: lessons from randomized trial. Ann Intern Med 1998;128:216–223.

14. RITA Trial Participants. Coronary angiography vs. coronary artery bypass surgery: the randomized Intervention Treatment of Angina (RITA) trial. Lancet 1993;341:573–580.

15. The BARI Investigators. Comparison of coronary artery bypass surgery with angioplasty in patients with multivessel disease. N Engl J Med 1996;335:217–225.

16. King SB III, Lembo NJ, Weintraub WS, et al. A randomized trial comparing coronary angioplasty with bypass surgery. N Engl J Med 1994;331:1044–1050.

17. Berkhoff D, Schmidt S, Schulman SP, et al. Transmyocardial laser revascularisation compared with continued medical therapy for treatment of refractory angino pectoris: a prospective randomized trial. Lancet 1999;354:885–890.

Chapter 8
Acute Coronary Syndrome

Patients with acute coronary syndrome (ACS) are characterized by having a multicentric, multivessel, generalized inflammatory process.

Q: How are the risks of acute coronary syndrome stratified?
Acute coronary syndrome is divided into unstable angina/non–ST-segment elevation MI (NSTEMI) and ST-segment elevation MI (STEMI) (Fig. 8.1).

RISK ASSESSMENT
A variety of factors may play a role, such as age, the severity of presenting symptoms, and other risk factors.[1] The features that indicate risk are as follows:

- High-mortality risks include age (>70 years), ST segment depression on the initial electrocardiogram (ECG), refractory angina, and recurrent ischemic symptoms not responding to treatment, markedly raised troponin, serious dysrhythmia, and left ventricular dysfunction (especially ejection fraction <40%). Patients with confirmed or suspected myocardial ischemia have a 50%, 10-year mortality, and those with NSTEMI have a 10-year mortality of 70%.[2]
- The medium risk is indicated by a positive history of MI or diabetes, mildly raised troponin, recurrent ischemia, left ventricular dysfunction, prolonged rest pain now relieved, and if patient is already taking aspirin. Elevated troponin (cTnl or cTnT) level, even in the presence of normal isoenzyme of creatine kinase with muscle and brain subunits (CK-MB) levels identify patients without ST-segment elevation who are at increased risk of death. The higher the troponin level, the greater the risk, but the rise needs to be sustained, not brief.
- Low-risk patients are younger, with no chest pain at rest, normal ECG, and negative troponin.

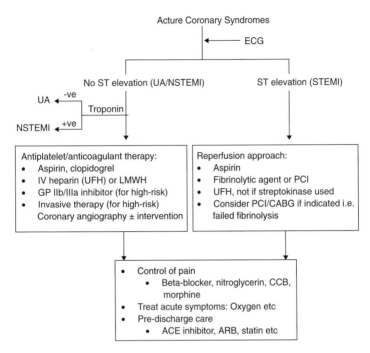

FIGURE 8.1. Acute coronary syndromes and their management strategies.

Recently it was observed that measurement of N-terminal probrain natriuretic peptide (NT-proBNP) in blood on admission improves the early risk stratification of patients in ACS.[3] CRP, heart rate and renal dysfunction also help. Antman et al developed a seven-point risk score, the 'TIMI Risk Score' (age ≥65 years, >3 coronary risk factors, prior angiographic obstruction, ST segment deviation, >2 angina events within 24 hours, use of aspirin with 7 days, and elevated cardiac markers).[4] The score was defined as the cumulative number of these variables, the risk of developing adverse outcome ranging from 5% with a score of 0–1 to 41% with a score of six or seven.

UNSTABLE ANGINA/NON–ST-SEGMENT ELEVATION MI

Unstable angina (UA) is responsible for up to 200,000 hospital admissions per year in the United Kingdom. Around 10% of unstable angina patients die or suffer a myocardial infarction (MI) within 6 months, despite the current best therapy with aspirin, heparin, and anticoagulants. In industrialized countries, the annual incidence of UA is around 6 per 10,000 in the general population.

Q: How does unstable angina differ from chronic stable angina?

Unstable angina is distinguished from stable angina, acute MI (AMI), and noncardiac pain by the pattern of symptoms (characteristic pain present at rest or on lower levels of activity), the severity of symptoms (recently increasing intensity, frequency, or duration). The chest pain comes on repeatedly, up to 20 times a day, and there is a 10% to 20% risk of heart attack. Unstable angina is due to the detachment of a stable clot or plaque from the wall of the coronary artery. This may cause spasm of the coronary artery, which results in myocardial ischemia, at least temporarily. Such a situation may also arise if a thrombus forms over the plaque or stenosis is worsened simply by coronary spasm. Unstable angina may also occur in association with other medical conditions, including heart valve disease, arrhythmia, and cardiomyopathy. Unstable angina falls between stable angina and heart attack in the wider spectrum of coronary artery disease (Fig. 8.2). Spasm of a diseased artery with a lumen already reduced by 25% may be enough to cause unstable angina. There could also be plaque fissuring. Unstable angina is classified according to the severity of symptoms (Table 8.1).

Key Features of Unstable Angina

- Angina at rest
- New-onset angina with a marked restriction in activity (walking 20–50 yards on a flat surface) in the preceding 4 to 8 weeks
- Angina of rapidly increasing severity, which is a changing pattern in a previously stable patient

Only one of the above criteria is required to make the diagnosis of unstable angina but all three may coexist.

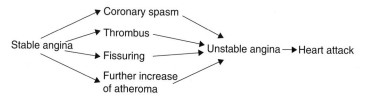

FIGURE 8.2. Interrelationship between stable and unstable angina and heart attack.

TABLE 8.1. Braunwald's classification of unstable angina (From Braunwald E., Unstable angina: a classification. Circulation 80(2):410–414, 1989)

Class	Features
	According to symptoms
I	New-onset, severe, or accelerated angina but no rest pain during the last 2 months
II	Sub-acute episode of angina during the preceding month but not within the previous 48 hours
III	Acute episode of angina at rest during preceding 48 hours; further classified into troponin-negative and troponin-positive types
	According to clinical circumstances
A	Angina develops in the presence of extracardiac conditions that intensifies myocardial ischemia
B	Primary unstable angina
C	Postmyocardial infarction unstable angina

Electrocardiographic Abnormalities

Electrocardiogram changes in UA/NSTEMI manifest as ST-segment depression and/or T-wave inversion, which may be transient (as in UA) or more persistent (as in NSTEMI). A normal ECG, however, does not exclude ACS. A deep symmetrical T wave in the anterior leads indicates proximal stenosis of the left anterior descending artery.

Q: What are the current views about the management of US/NSTEMI?

All patients with the diagnosis of ACS should be admitted to the coronary care unit. Patients with unstable angina require deactivation of platelets and dissolution of the thrombus and relief of myocardial ischemic symptoms. The main strategy is the antithrombotic approach.

Reduction of Myocardial Demand/Antiischemic Treatment

This aspect of management of ACS (UA and NSTEMI) is essentially the same as for angina, except that it is more aggressive. Nitrates, beta-blockers, diltiazem, and verapamil are used in unstable angina. Nitrates are useful for pain management in acute ischemia and should initially be given sublingually or orally. If pain becomes worse, nitrates are given intravenously. Beta-blockers are given to all who do not have contraindications; otherwise calcium channel blockers (CCBs), such as diltiazem is given. Diltiazem may reduce the risk of reinfarction in patients with non–Q-wave infarction. In patients with rest pain or those at high risk, an initial intravenous dose of atenolol or metoprolol of 5 mg over 2 minutes, and then a further 5 mg after 10 minutes, should be given. Intravenous beta-blocker is indicated where rapid action is required in patients with continuing angina, with tachycardia but without heart failure or hypertension. Oral treatment is sufficient for lower-risk patients.

Dihydropyridine calcium antagonists, such as nifedipine, should not be given alone in unstable angina. Trials with short-acting nifedipine suggested a trend to increased risk of MI or recurrent ischemia. However, when nifedipine is added to a beta-blocker for patients with continuing pain, symptom relief is improved. The potassium-channel opener nicorandil was recently shown to produce symptomatic benefit in patients whose pain was uncontrolled by maximal dosages of other antianginal agents.

Antithrombotic Therapy

The purpose of antithrombotic therapy including antiplatelets and anticoagulants is to prevent progression of thrombus and to facilitate its lysis. Antiplatelet therapy with aspirin, clopidogrel (or ticlopidine) and glycoprotein (GP) IIb/IIIa antagonist have been found useful in the management of unstable angina. All patients should take aspirin, 300 mg and clopidogrel, 300 mg stat, followed with 75–160 mg daily of aspirin indefinitely as a maintenance dose and clopidogrel, 75 mg for up to 9 months. If a patient is allergic, then clopidogrel alone should be prescribed, as it is a suitable alternative.[5] In the RISC study, low-dose oral aspirin (75 mg daily) reduced the risk of heart attack or death after an episode of unstable ACS by 50% at 3 months.[6] Aspirin reduces death and progression to MI in patients with unstable angina by 30%.[7] Co-prescribing clopidogrel with aspirin in unstable angina effects a modest reduction in nonfatal MI, but increases the risk of bleeding.[8] If aspirin resistance is suspected, clopidogrel should be added and aspirin not discontinued.

The final common pathway of platelet aggregation is the GP IIb/IIIa receptor, through which activated platelets adhere to each other; GP IIb/IIIa receptor antagonists are potent inhibitors of platelet aggregation. There are three GP IIb/IIIa receptor antagonists: abciximab, eptifibatide, and tirofiban. A meta-analysis of 16 randomized controlled trials confirmed that these agents have modest beneficial effects (relative risk reduction of 14%) in patients during PCTA of ACS.[9] Abciximab does not appear to be beneficial in patients with unstable angina without the context of percutaneous coronary intervention. When using GP IIb/IIIa, the dose of heparin needs to be reduced. If bleeding occurs, GP IIb/IIIa should be stopped.

Thrombolytic (Fibrinolytic) Therapy

Unlike AMI, patients without ST-segment elevation (UA and NSTEMI) do not benefit from immediate aggressive thrombolytic therapy. Thrombolytic therapy is not recommended for US/NSTEMI patients. It may in fact harm them.

ACC/AHA Guidelines for Antithrombotic Therapy in UA/NSTEMI[10]

CLASS I

1. Aspirin should be given immediately and continued indefinitely.

2. Clopidogrel is given to hospitalized patients who are unable to take aspirin.

3. In hospitalized patients in whom an early noninterventional approach is planned, clopidogrel should be added to aspirin immediately for at least 1 month and given up to 9 months.

4. GP IIb/IIIa antagonist should be added to aspirin and heparin in patients in whom catheterization and percutaneous coronary intervention (PCI) are planned.

5. In patients taking clopidogrel in whom elective CABG is planned, the drug would be withheld for 5 to 7 days.

6. Intravenous UFH or subcutaneous LMWH should be added to antiplatelet therapy with aspirin and/or clopidogrel.

CLASS IIa

1. Eptifibatide or tirofiban should be given in addition to aspirin, low-molecular-weight heparin (LMWH), or unfractionated heparin (UFH) to patients with continuing ischemic symptoms, an elevated troponin, or with other high-risk features in whom an invasive management strategy is not planned.

2. A platelet GP IIb/IIIa inhibitor should be given to patients already receiving heparin, aspirin, or clopidogrel in whom catheterization and PCI are planned.

Antithrombin Agents

These agents include heparin, LMWH, and hirudin. Anticoagulation with heparin should be started as soon as possible, if there is no contraindication. Heparin (i.e., unfractionated heparin) is a heterogeneous mucopolysaccharide that binds antithrombin, which increases the inhibition of thrombin and factor Xa. The benefit of using unfractionated heparin in unstable angina is well established. A meta-analysis showed that in addition to aspirin, intravenous heparin provided a relative risk reduction of 33% in the risk of death or MI.[11] Its disadvantage is that it has unpredictable anticoagulant effect. It is, however, cheap, relatively reliable, and reversible.

LMWH is a subfraction of standard heparin and it has number of benefits over UFH. These include the potential to prevent thrombin generation as well as inhibit thrombin, no need to monitor with coagulation testing, a lower rate of heparin-associated thrombocytopenia, and its ability to be administered subcutaneously. However, the disadvantage is that its action cannot be easily reversed if the need arises, such as in patients who are likely to have an emergency revascularization procedure. In those patients, to avoid this problem, UFH should be used, which has an equivalent benefit, but with enoxaparin, the benefit is greater.[12] GP IIb/IIIa inhibitor can be used with LMWH.

Conclusion

Low-risk cases may be managed by taking aspirin, clopidogrel, a beta-blocker (e.g., atenolol 50 to 100 mg orally daily) with or without a CCBs (diltiazem, verapamil) and isosorbide mononitrate. They are assessed using the treadmill test. Intermediate and high-risk patients are assessed by early coronary angiography. They need intensive therapy with beta-blockers, aspirin, clopidrogel, LMWH, and GP IIb/IIIa inhibitors.

Coronary artery bypass grafting is recommended for most patients with left main artery disease or for many with three-vessel disease in the presence of impairment of left ventricular function. Alternatively, some may need angioplasty. Angioplasty and stenting, with appropriate use of antiplatelet agents such as abciximab, are ideally suited for single-vessel disease. In unstable angina patients with single-vessel disease, success rates of 80% to 90% can be achieved in patients with suitable anatomy. Coronary stent insertion increases the effectiveness of short- and mid-term angioplasty in unstable angina. More than 90% of unstable angina will stabilize with maximal medical treatment; for those who do not stabilize, coronary angiography is indicated.

Long-Term Management of Unstable Angina

The long-term patient should follow the same treatment advised for secondary prevention. These patients should be on aspirin indefinately and clopidrogel for at least 9 months unless contraindicated. Lipid-lowering drugs should be prescribed as they have a significant effect on the morphology of plaque. The Myocardial Ischemia Reduction with Aggressive Cholesterol Lowering

(MIRACL) Trial showed that intensive cholesterol lowering with atorvastatin immediately after hospitalization for unstable angina or NSTEMI reduced the incidence of recurrent ischemic over the next 4 months.[13] A fibrate or niacin should be used if HDL-C is <40 mg/dl (1.0 mmol/L), as an isolated finding or with other lipid abnormalities. Angiotensin-converting enzyme (ACE) inhibitor should be used, as its benefit goes beyond blood pressure control and may relate to plaque stabilization.

ACUTE MYOCARDIAL INFARCTION (STEMI)

Each year, about 900,000 people in the United States suffer AMI, about 225,000 of whom die. More than 60% of the deaths occur within 1 hour of the attack and are attributable to arrhythmias, mostly ventricular fibrillation. AMI is one of the most common causes of mortality in developing and developed countries. Non-atheromatous coronary artery disease (CAD) may be due to congenital abnormalities in the origin or distribution of coronary arteries. The most common anomalies are the following:

1. The abnormal origin of a coronary artery (usually the left) from the pulmonary artery, origin of both coronary arteries from the right or left sinus of Valsalva, and arteriovenous fistula.
2. Anomalous origin of either the left main coronary artery or right coronary artery from the aorta with subsequent coursing between the aorta and pulmonary trunk.
3. Dissection of a coronary artery.
4. Inherited connective tissue disorders, which are associated with myocardial ischemia, include Marfan syndrome, Hurler syndrome, homocystinuria, and Ehlers-Danlos syndrome (coronary artery dissection), etc.
5. Myocardial ischemia due to embolism, implanted prosthetic valves, primary tumors of the heart, emboli from mural thrombus.

Q: What is the clinical presentation of AMI and what are its complications?

Acute myocardial infarction (AMI) can be defined, as a condition in which there is myocardial necrosis caused by acute interruptions of coronary blood supply. Myocardial infarction usually starts with erosion, cracking, or rupture of an atheromatous plaque in the coronary artery. This causes platelet aggregaton and activation, leading to thrombus formation. Complete occlusion of the coronary artery finally ensues and this results in myocardial ischemia, which may be made worse by coronary spasm or embolism of platelets distally, causing arrhythmia or cardiac arrest. Cardiac ischemia causes chest pain, similar to that of angina but of greater intensity and longer duration. It is also responsible for electrocardiographic changes (e.g., ST elevation, bundle branch block) noticed over ischemic area. These electrocardiographic changes may be delayed or may not occur. If ischemia persists, the cardiac muscle may infarct, which appears on the ECG as development of Q waves (Q-wave infarction) and causes a rise of cardiac enzymes (e.g., creatine kinase [CK]) and of cardiac troponin T and I. Prompt administration of thrombolytic therapy or angioplasty in these patients facilitates restoration of normal coronary blood flow, and this may reverse ST elevation and prevent or limit infarction. Myocardial infarction may be transmural, when the whole thickness of the ventricular wall is necrosed or subendocardial (nontransmural), when the necrosis involves the subendocardium only.

Precipitating Factors
The peak incidence of AMI and sudden cardiac death is at about 9 a.m. The early morning hours are associated with rises in plasma catecholamines and cortisol and increased platelet aggregability. A significant number of AMIs occur within few hours of severe physical exertion, and could be the result of marked increase in myocardial oxygen consumption in the presence of severe coronary arterial narrowing. Exertion or mental stress may trigger plaque disruption. Other precipitating factors of AMI include respiratory infections/embolism, hypoxia, hypoglycemia, reduced myocardial perfusion, secondary serum sickness, and a wasp sting. However, 50% cases have no known cause.

Atypical Presentations
In 20% to 60% of cases, AMI is first detected at a routine ECG findings or at postmortem examination. Of these about half are silent, and these are more common in patients with hypertension and diabetes. Silent infarction is often followed by silent ischemia. In the other half, the patient is able to recall symptoms suggestive of MI when questioned. Atypical presentation includes silent MI, congestive heart failure, classical angina, atypical site of pain, cerebral vascular insufficiency, acute indigestion, and extreme lethargy.

Physical Findings
The patient with AMI is often anxious, restless, breathless, gasping, and has pallor. Blood-stained frothy sputum may be coughed. There may be signs of cardiogenic shock. There is often tachycardia of 100 to 110 per minute, but the rate may vary from brady-

cardia to severe tachycardia. The rhythm is usually regular initially, though premature ventricular beats appear in most patients. Systolic blood pressure and pulse pressure are usually reduced. Initially, the blood pressure may be elevated >160/90 mm Hg, possibly due to adrenergic discharge secondary to pain and agitation. The blood pressure usually falls progressively during the first week and returns to normal in 2 to 3 weeks. There may be sudden severe hypotension. There is mild to moderate elevation of temperature, which settles by the end of week. The jugular venous pressure is usually normal or slightly elevated in the early course of AMI.

The examination of the heart may be normal despite severe AMI, but frequently a presystolic pulsation, synchronous with an audible fourth heart sound, is present. The signs of left ventricular dysfunction may be noted. There is often slight leukocytosis and an increase in the erythrocyte sedimentation rate (ESR).

Differential Diagnosis

The diagnosis of AMI mainly depends on clinical features, ECG changes, and biochemical markers of myocardial injury. AMI should be differentiated from other causes of chest pain, such as pleurisy, pulmonary embolism, dissection of the aorta, pericarditis, myocarditis, esophagitis, peptic ulcer, pancreatitis, herpes zoster, and nerve root lesion.

Complications

Complications do not follow every heart attack, but the first 48 hours are very critical. The following are the common complications:

Disorders of Conduction

Almost 95% of cases with AMI develop some kind of disorder of conduction, rhythm, or rate. Half of these are severe enough to be of clinical importance. Arrhythmias that commonly complicate AMI include sinus bradycardia, sinus tachycardia, atrial premature beats, atrial fibrillation, ventricular premature beats, ventricular tachycardia, ventricular fibrillation, and atrioventricular block. However, ventricular fibrillation (VF) causes the most concern and is the most frequent single cause of death. In minutes preceding primary ventricular fibrillation, there is often an increase in the frequency and complexity of ventricular ectopy and that of proximal ventricular tachycardia. The greatest risk of sudden death after AMI is in the first 6 to 12 hours. Further tests may be useful to assess the presence of residual myocardial ischemia, functional status (exercise testing), and ventricular function. Holter monitoring may help to detect proximal ventricular ectopics and ventricular arrhythmia.

Other Complications

Congestive heart failure may develop in 24 to 48 hours in 75% of cases of AMI. Despite all treatment, 70% of patients with cardiogenic shock die. Rupture of cardiac wall or a septum is a rare complication. Rupture of the papillary muscle leads to mitral regurgitation. Ventricular aneurysm is rare but serious. Postinfarction ischemia has been noticed in approximately 20% to 30% of patients. It is a bad prognostic sign, and these patients frequently need catherization to assess for PCI. Pericarditis is a direct consequence of the underlying myocardial damage and usually resolves in a week. It is a common cause of persistent chest pain in the first 3 days following transmural MI. About 40% of patients develop Dressler's syndrome, which clinically presents as fever, often with pericarditis and pleurisy, 2 to 12 weeks after AMI. The incidence of deep vein thrombosis (DVT) or pulmonary embolism is drastically reduced due to early mobilization. However, if it occurs, it needs anticoagulation.

Q: What is the diagnostic and prognostic value of different biochemical cardiac markers in AMI?

Biochemical markers of myocardial damage are useful for confirming the diagnosis of AMI, when the patient presents without ST-segment elevation, when the diagnosis is unclear, and when the physician must distinguish patients with unstable angina from those with a non–Q-wave MI. Serum cardiac enzymes also provide valuable prognostic information and help to plan management. The three classical myocardial markers that are still used are creatine kinase (CK), aspartate transaminase (AST), and lactic dehydrogenase (LDH). The serum LDH level in the blood is increased by 12 to 18 hours after the onset of AMI, reaches peak at 48 to 72 hours, and returns to normal in 6 to 10 days (Fig. 8.3). The serum AST level rises above normal 8 to 12 hours after AMI, peaks at 24 to 36 hours, and returns to normal in 3 to 5 days. The newer markers are classical enzyme CK-MB and completely new cardiac markers (i.e., the troponins).

Creatine Kinase

Creatine kinase (CK) is composed of three isoenzymes: CK-BB (CK-1), CK-MB (CK-2), and CK-MM (CK-3). CK-BB is found mainly in kidneys and brain, CK-MM is predominantly found in

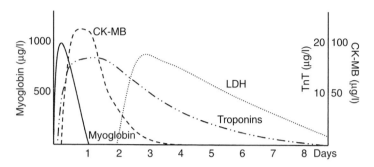

FIGURE 8.3. Evolution of serum biomarkers in acute myocardial infarction.

skeletal muscles, and CK-MB is predominantly found in the cardiac muscle but is also present in the uterus and placenta. CK-MB levels are also raised in thyroid, prostate, and lung cancers. In the absence of injury to these tissues, elevation of CK-MB is highly suggestive of AMI. Since CK-MB comprises 1% to 3% in the skeletal muscles, any trauma to skeletal muscle can raise CK-MB level in the blood. Therefore, to make a diagnosis of AMI from the estimation of CK-MB, it is a common practice to calculate the ratio of CK-MB/total CK; >2.5% indicates myocardial damage when using the sensitive monoclonal ("mass") assay.

Various biochemical tests measure CK and its isoforms. These tests comprise total CK, CK-MB, CK mass, and CK isoforms. The isoenzyme of CK (CK-BB, CK-MB, and CK-MM) have a number of isoforms. These increase the diagnostic sensitivity of CK-MB. There is only one isoform of CK-MB and CK-MM in the myocardium (CK-MB-2 and CK-MM-3). Isoforms of CK-MB are more sensitive than CK and CK-MB during the early stages of AMI.[14] CK-MB exists only in one form in myocardial tissue but in different isoforms in the plasma. An absolute level of CK-MB-2 >1 U/l or a ratio of CK-MB-2 to CK-MB-1 of 1.5 has improved sensitivity and specificity for the diagnosis of AMI within the first 6 hours as compared to conventional CK-MB.

The total CK level begins to rise between 6 and 12 hours after the onset of AMI, and peaks at 12 to 24 hours. CK-MB, however, starts to rise early, within 3 to 8 hours, peaks 8 to 58 (usually 24) hours, and returns to normal within 48 to 72 hours. CK and MB isoenzymes lack sufficient sensitivity and specificity. It is estimated that about 30% of patients presenting without ST-segment elevation who would otherwise be diagnosed with unstable angina are actually suffering a non–Q-wave MI when assessed with cardiac specific troponin measurements, because troponins are more sensitive.

Troponins

Troponin (Tn) is a regulatory protein in muscle cells that controls interactions between myosin and actin. It has three subunits, TnC, TnI, and TnT, which are found in skeletal and cardiac muscle. cTnI and cTnT are virtually absent from blood, and even minor elevation is indicative of myocyte damage. Troponin is therefore a highly sensitive and specific marker of myocardial damage, and some studies suggest that TnT 10 hours post-pain is 100% sensitive.[14–16] Troponin is released within 3 to 4 hours of injury, peaking after 12–24 hours, and remains detectable for up to 14 days (up to 7 days for cTnI and 10 days for cTnT). As troponin remains elevated for 2 weeks or so, the diagnosis of reinfarction within that period is difficult, unless concomitant measurements of CK-MB are done. Elevated cTnI or cTnT levels, in the presence of normal CK-MB, identify patients who derive greater benefit from GP IIb/IIIa inhibitor than patients without elevated troponin. An elevated troponin T has a predictive value for myocardial ischemia several times higher than that of CK-MB mass. Troponins are useful in identifying patients with AMI even in the absence of ST elevation. Elevated troponin cTnI or cTnT provides more prognostic information. Patients with negative troponin levels are at low risk, and those with elevated levels are at increased risk. The higher the level of troponin, the greater the risk. Patients with elevated troponin at <6 hours from the onset of pain have an increased risk of death.

Myoglobin

Myoglobin is a small-heme protein found in cardiac and skeletal muscles. It is more sensitive than CK-MB in AMI but not specific to cardiac damage. It is released in 1 to 3 hours, peaking at 4 to 8 hours, and returns to normal in 24 hours. CK-MB subforms are most efficient for early diagnosis (within 6 hours) of AMI, whereas cTnI and cTnT are highly specific and particularly effective for the late diagnosis for AMI. For the diagnosis of AMI within 2 or 3 hours of onset of symptoms, measurement of myoglobin and CK-MB subforms is suitable.

Electrocardiogram (ECG)

A pathological Q wave indicates MI but does not indicate if it is due to a new MI or to one suffered previously, ST and T segment changes help to distinguish them. Q-wave infarction has a different ECG evolution with ST-segment elevation, reciprocal ST-segment depression, and ultimate T-wave inversion and appearance of Q waves. Non–Q-wave infarction, on the other hand, may not produce any significant ECG changes or show only minor ST-segment depression. In non–Q-wave changes, there is less mortality, but there may be more risk of postinfarction angina.[17]

The sequence of ECG changes following AMI comprise an increase in amplitude of the T wave in leads facing the infracted ventricle. Within minutes this is accompanied by a significant ST-segment elevation, curving upward and englobing the T wave. The R wave, which initially increases in voltage in leads facing the infracted area, soon decreases, the T wave inverts and the Q wave develops. After a period of a few days or weeks, the abnormalities consist of a large Q wave and symmetrically inverted T waves. Following reperfusion, the ST segment returns to normal quickly; otherwise it takes several hours to several days or even longer if a myocardial scar has developed. The T wave remains inverted or becomes flat. (Fig. 8.4).

Usually ST elevation indicates myocardial injury, while QRS changes are due to transmural necrosis. In most patients initial elevation of the ST segment falls, during the first 12 hours, followed by a plateau, and it finally becomes normal in a few days but the T wave remains inverted. An abnormal Q wave develops and the R-wave loss occurs as early as 2 hours after the onset of pain, and these changes are fully developed within 4 to 14 hours. Weeks and

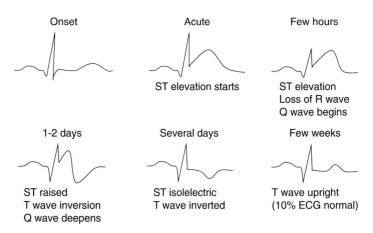

FIGURE 8.4. Evolution of ECG changes following acute transmural myocardial infarction.

months following AMI, the ST segment and T wave have often returned to normal, but a pathological Q wave persists. The ECG changes appear more rapidly in inferior than anterior myocardial infarction. These changes occur in leads overlying the zone of infarction (Table 8.2). The reciprocal changes are observed in the corresponding leads opposite to that site. For instance, in anteroseptal MI, ST-segment elevation occurs in V1 and V2, the reciprocal changes of ST-segment depression, then occur in the leads opposite (i.e., inferior, LII, III, aVF). Pathological Q waves have a width of at least the size of a small box and a depth of greater than 25% of the total height of the QRS complex. They appear in the leads overlying the infarction zone.

Other Diagnostic Tests

An X-ray of the chest may reveal signs of left ventricular failure and cardiomegaly. Computed tomography (CT) can provide useful cross-sectional information such as assessment of cavity dimensions, wall thickness, and left ventricular aneurysm. Various forms of cardiac imaging—radionuclide, angiography, perfusion scintigraphy, and positron emission tomography—are used in the diagnosis of AMI. Magnetic resonance imaging (MRI) can detect AMI and assesses the severity of the ischemic insult. However, a patient who is acutely ill cannot be transported to an MRI unit, but echocardiographic equipment can be easily moved to the patient; therefore, it is an invaluable technique used in critically ill, hospitalized patients in the diagnosis of AMI where ECG findings were equivocal or nondiagnostic.

TABLE 8.2. ECG changes and site of lesion in acute myocardial infarction

MI sites	Leads	ECG	Site of lesion
Inferior	II, III, aVL	Q, ST, T	RCA
Lateral	I, aVL, V_5, V_6	Q, ST, T	Circumflex, branch of LCA
Anterior	V_1–V_6, I, aVL	Q, ST, T, loss of R	Interventricular branch of LCA
Posterior	V_1, V_2	R > S, ST depression elevated T	RCA
Anterioseptal	V_1, V_2, V_3	Q, ST, T, loss of R in V_1	LAD

RCA, right coronary artery; LCA, left coronary artery; LAD, left anterior descending artery; Q, Q wave; ST, ST elevation; T, T inversion; R > S, fall T waves.

Q: What are the essential steps in the management of acute myocardial infarction?

The main keys to managing the patients with myocardial infarction are relief of pain, early hospital admission to enable detection of arrhythmias and their treatment, and institution of reperfusion approach. Thrombolytic therapy, aspirin, statin, and ACE inhibitors may favorably influence the outcome in a patient with AMI. Aspirin and intravenous beta-blockers are shown to improve outcome when given acutely.[18] Aspirin, ACE inhibitors, beta-blockers, and coumarin anticoagulants in post-MI cases have been shown to reduce the risk of further cardiovascular morbidity and mortality and improve survival. The following factors are important in the management of AMI:

Oxygen

Oxygen should be administered to all AMI patients who have clinical signs of arterial hypoxemia or if it can be confirmed by measurement (SaO_2 <90%). There is general agreement about giving oxygen to all patients with uncomplicated AMI during the first 2 to 3 hours, but there is some conflicting evidence about giving oxygen beyond 3 to 6 hours. Oxygen should be given in just sufficient doses for 24 to 84 hours (100% oxygen at 2 to 4 L/min). Serial arterial oxygen estimation should be performed in all AMI. Pulsed oximetry should be done as a routine.

ECG

A 12-lead ECG should be recorded in all patients. If it is normal and the symptoms persist, frequent ECG or continuous ST-segment monitoring should be performed.

Blood Tests

Blood tests should include markers of cardiac damage, high-sensitivity C-reactive protein (hsCRP), and ESR. Serial biomarkers are useful in assessing the success of reperfusion of the infarcted artery after fibrinolytic therapy, and it is also of prognostic value.

Imaging

Imaging should be done in all cases, but it should not delay reperfusion therapy unless aortic dissection is suspected; then echocardiography, contrast CT scan, or MRI may have diagnostic value. However, in selected patients portable echocardiography is reasonable to do for diagnostic and prognostic reasons.

Thrombolytic Therapy

In patients presenting within 12 hours of onset of symptoms with ST elevation or left bundle branch block on the initial ECG, thrombolytic therapy is given immediately without waiting for the results of cardiac markers, if not already given before admission (by ambulance staff). Even if ECG is normal, reperfusion therapy should not be delayed. Thrombolytics should ideally be given within 6 hours of onset of symptoms, but patients may still benefit if it is administered at between 6 and 12 hours in high-risk patients such as large anterior infarcts. The evidence suggests that it is far more important to give any thrombolytic promptly rather than to debate which one should be used. Thrombolytics have not been proven to help patients whose ECG is normal or shows only ST depression, or who present over 12 hours after symptom onset. Thrombolysis is further discussed later in this chapter.

Heparin and GP IIb/IIIa

For patients with AMI already on aspirin, there is a lack of published direct evidence that routine use of IV or SC heparin (with or without thrombolytic therapy) confers a clinical advantage. Heparin is useful in maintaining vessel patency. Experiments show that heparin increases the thrombolytic potential of tissue-type plasminogen activator (tPA). UFH should be given to patients undergoing a revascularization procedure, reperfusion with alteplase, reteplase, or tenecteplase; and those patients treated with nonselective fibrinolytic agents (streptokinase, anistreplase, or urokinase) who are at high risk for systemic emboli (large or anterior MI, atrial fibrillation, previous thrombus, known left ventricular thrombus, or cardiogenic shock). LMWH might be considered as an alternative to UFH with perfusion therapy in patients less than 75 years of age, provided there is no significant renal impairment. Enoxaparin used with full-dose tenecteplase is the most comprehensively studied regimen in patients under 75 years of age.[19] For a patient who is known to have heparin-induced thrombocytopenia, it is reasonable to consider bivalirudin as an alternative to heparin to be used in conjunction with streptokinase. Where more effective thrombolysis is needed, a combined low-dose tPA with full-dose GP IIb/IIIa inhibitors can be used.

Nitrates

So long as the patient does not suffer from hypotension (i.e., systolic BP <100 mm Hg or a decline of >25 mm Hg from the patient's previous normal blood pressure), sublingual nitroglycerin can be given in the dose of 0.4 mg every 5 minutes up to three doses. The patient should be closely monitored for the vital signs and BP. The use of intravenous nitroglycerin should be assessed. Intravenous nitroglycerin is indicated for the relief of continuing ischemic discomfort, control of hypertension, and pulmonary congestion. Nitroglycerin should not be given to patients who have taken phosphodiesterase inhibitor during the last 24 hours (48 hours for tadalafil). Use of nitrates should be avoided in inferior wall infarction due to the risk of sudden hypotension and bradycardia. However, if this situation has risen, giving atropine intravenously could reverse it. Nitrates may relieve ischemic chest pain and symptoms of left ventricular failure, and may have some antiaggregatory action on platelets. There is no definite proof that nitrates given for 4 to 6 weeks post-MI increase survival. Long-acting nitrates can be started after stopping intravenous nitrates. IV nitroglycerine is given in the dose of 10 μg/min initially, titrated every 20–30 minutes by 20 μg/min to a maximum 400 μg/min. IV isosorbide is given initially in a dose of 2 mg/hour up to 10 mg/hour if necessary.

Analgesics

Pain relief in AMI is the most important first step. Since the pain in AMI is due to ischemia, any intervention that improves the oxygen supply–demand relationship may relieve pain. Morphine sulphate (2–4 mg IV with increments of 2–8 mg IV repeated at 5- to 10-minute interval) at the rate of 1 mg per minute should be given. Metoclopramide 10 mg IV should be given with morphine to prevent nausea and vomiting. IV beta-blockers, thrombolytics, and nitrates all relieve pain by limiting ischemic changes.

Antiplatelet Agents

Aspirin 162 to 325 mg should be chewed immediately and continued daily indefinitely in the dose of 75 to 162 mg. If patient has not already taken this before hospital admission, it should be given in the hospital as soon as possible. Slow-release or buffered forms of aspirin should be avoided. However, aspirin suppository (325 mg) can be used by those who suffer nausea, vomiting, or upper gastrointestinal tract symptoms. Other antiplatelet agents, such as clopidogrel and ticlopidine, can be used if the patient is allergic to or intolerant of aspirin.

The International Study of Infarct Survival (ISIS-2) has shown conclusively the efficacy of aspirin alone for the treatment of AMI, with a 35-day mortality reduction of 23%, when combined with either streptokinase or alteplase.[20] In the group of patients randomly assigned to receive aspirin alone, there was a 23% reduction in mortality, whereas in the group assigned to receive intravenous streptokinase alone, there was a 23% reduction. The benefit in survival conferred by aspirin was additive to that with streptokinase; the in-hospital combination of aspirin and streptokinase reduced mortality by 42%. Also, nonfatal strokes and reinfarction were reduced in the aspirin-treated groups in the ISIS-2 study. The efficacy of low-dose aspirin in coronary thrombosis is not assessed.

Use of Aspirin vs. Clopidogrel Post-MI

A randomized, blinded trial of clopidogrel versus aspirin in patients at risk of ischemic events has shown that clopidogrel is a suitable alternative to aspirin.[5] After a mean follow-up period of 1.9 years, the annual risk of the combined outcome of ischemic stroke, myocardial infarction, or vascular death in the clopidogrel-treated group was 5.32% compared to 5.83% in the aspirin-treated group. The data suggested a very small but statistically significant benefit of clopidogrel over aspirin in the prevention of further vascular events and vascular deaths in patients with established atherosclerosis including that of post-MI. Clopidogrel combined with aspirin is recommended in AMI patients who undergo stent insertion.

Beta-Blockers

An oral beta-blocker should be given to all patients without contraindication irrespective of concomitant fibrinolytic therapy or performance of percutaneous intervention. It is reasonable to give a beta-blocker intravenously in AMI patients without contraindication, especially if the patient has tachyarrhythmia or hypertension. An intravenous beta-blocker reduces pain, recurrent ischemia, and mortality in AMI patients, with a two- to threefold reduction in the risk of cardiac rupture,[21] and most of those advantages are obtained by using them in the first 24 hours. Metoprolol and atenolol can be given intravenously slowly in the dose of 5 mg initially and repeated after 5 minutes while the patient is being monitored. The heart rate should not drop below 50/min and systolic BP below 100 mm Hg. These drugs relieve pain, lessen the need of analgesics, and limit the size of the infarct by reducing ischemia. The long-term use of beta-blocker post-MI is well established. Their use post-MI is described later in this chapter.

Angiotensin-Converting Enzyme (ACE) Inhibitors and Angiotensin Receptor Blockers (ARBs)

Angiotensin-converting enzyme inhibitors should be given orally within 24 hours of AMI (after fibrinolytic therapy has been completed and BP stabilized) to patients with anterior infarct, pulmonary congestion, or left ventricular (LV) ejection fraction ≤40% in the absence of hypotension. Angiotensin receptor blockers should be prescribed to patients who are intolerant of ACE inhibitors, have LV ejection fraction ≤40%, or have diabetes or heart failure. These drugs are discussed later in this chapter. Valsartan and candesartan have demonstrated the efficacy of this recommendation.[10]

Reperfusion
All patients should have reperfusion (fibrinolysis or PCI). It is discussed elsewhere in this chapter.

Other Therapies
Patients with frequent premature ventricular ectopics do better with prophylactic antiarrhythmic drugs such as amiodarone, but routine prophylactic antiarrhythmic therapy (e.g., flecanide, amiodarone, quinidine, or lidocaine) appear not to reduce, and may increase, mortality rates in AMI. Coumarin anticoagulants in post-MI are also associated with a reduced risk of reinfarction, coronary death, and stroke. Coumarins are reserved for those patients who suffered large anterior infarction, left ventricular aneurysm, paroxysmal tachycardia, chronic heart failure, and systemic embolic disease. The routine use of anticoagulants in AMI is controversial, but it is indicated in preventing DVT and left ventricular thrombi, and possibly in the limitation of infarct. Long-term anticoagulation is useful for secondary prevention following AMI in high-risk patients. The Warfarin Reinfarction Study (WARIS) reported a 50% reduction in combined outcomes of recurrent infarction, stroke, and mortality.[22] Similarly, the anticoagulants in the secondary prevention of events in coronary thrombosis (ASPECT) trial reported ≥50% reduction in reinfarction and a 40% reduction in stroke among survivors of MI.[23] Each study found an increased incidence of bleeding with anticoagulants.[23] Diabetes needs to be strictly controlled, as these patients have a 50% greater risk of reinfarction. An insulin infusion to normalize blood sugar is recommended for patients with AMI. A randomized controlled trial involving 620 patients with diabetes mellitus and AMI compared conventional therapy (i.e., using insulin only where clinically indicated) with intensive insulin therapy (i.e., IV insulin-glucose infusion for at least 24 hours, followed by subcutaneous dose four times daily for at least 3 months).[24] Mortality rates were lower in the intensive-insulin group, both at 1 year (19% vs. 26%) and at 3.4

years (33% vs. 44%). Intensive therapy with lipid-lowering drugs should be considered for all hospitalized patients for ACS. The optimal goal should be <70 mg/dl (1.8 mmol/dl). The choice of drugs and dosage should be guided in part by measurement of LDL-C within 24 hours of admission to the hospital. Therapy can be modified at follow-up, if necessary. There is no place of magnesium in post MI patients.[33]

Methods Useful in Estimating the Size of an Infarct[19]
- Serial ECG changes: All patients should have an ECG at 24 hours and at discharge to assess the success of reperfusion and the extent of infarction (presence or absence of new Q wave).
- Serial creatine kinase and the creatine kinase-MB isoenzyme are most widely accepted to estimate the size of infarct.
- Radionuclide imaging with technetium-sestamibi (single photon emission computed tomography [SPECT] approach).
- Echochardiography helps in the assessment of global and regional left ventricular function.
- Magnetic resonance imaging provides good estimation of both the transmural and circumferential extent of infarction.

Q: What are the advantages of one thrombolytic drug over another?
Thrombolytic drugs activate plasminogen, which degrades fibrin and breaks down thrombi. Thrombolysis has a beneficial effect in all cases, but more marked in patients with anterior MI, diabetes, low blood pressure (<100 mm Hg systolic), or tachycardia (>100 heart beats per minute). The earlier the treatment is started, the more beneficial it is. The greatest benefit is obtained if the thrombolytic is started within 3 hours of onset of pain. Coronary thrombolysis helps to restore coronary patency, preserves left ventricular function, and improves survival.

The three main thrombolytic drugs are streptokinase, recombinant tissue type plasminogen activator (alteplase, tPA), reteplase (rPA), and tenecteplase (TNK-tPA). Streptokinase (and urokinase) act by stimulating the activator of endogenous plasminogen to plasmin. Plasmin achieves thrombolysis by breaking the fibrin directly. The conversion of plasminogen also takes place in the systemic circulation, so hemorrhage may occur. Antibodies are also produced against streptokinase, so treatment should not be repeated within 12 months. Streptokinase is given in the dose of 1.5 million units over 1 hour. The newer plasminogen activators (e.g., tPA, rPA, TNK-tPA/tenecteplase) are genetically engineered versions of the naturally occurring tissue plasminogen activator.

They differ from streptokinase (and urokinase) in that they bind preferentially to fibrin in a formed thrombus, thereby generating plasmin locally within the coronary arteries, with less disturbance of fibrinogen in the general circulation. They should have a greater effect than streptokinase on coronary artery patency, which should provide better clinical outcome. Because they are the products of recombinant DNA technology, there should be no allergic reaction, therefore enabling their use repeatedly. As rPA and TNK-tPA are mutants of tPA with longer lives, their other advantage is that they can be given as a bolus rather than IV infusion, unlike tPA and streptokinase. Reteplase, a modified plasminogen activator, is produced to overcome some of the limitations of tPA by having an increased resistance to breakdown. It has been introduced as an alternative to tPA, as has TNK-tPA. But unfortunately, patency rates have been shown to be no better with reteplase. Lanoteplase and saruplase (a recombinant urokinase plasminogen activator) have not been shown to be superior to tPA.

The benefit of coronary thrombolytics is clearly noted, independently from sex, BP and heart rate on admission, history of previous MI, diabetes, and age. The benefit was also manifested in the older age group (>75 years). A clear and major benefit was seen in patients with ST segment elevation on ECG and bundle branch block, because 90% of these patients showed total coronary occlusion by an intracoronary thrombus. No difference in the mortality rate of three thrombolytic agents (alteplase, stretokinase, anisolylated plasminogen streptokinase activator complex) was noted. More strokes, particularly hemorrhagic types, occurred with tPA than with streptokinase.[25,26] However, combining death and strokes, there was still a benefit favoring tPA (6.9% vs. 7.8%).[27] Decreasing ST-segment depression in ECG and a rapid peak in myoglobin in the blood are indicators of successful thrombolysis.

Risks and Contraindications
Thrombolytic therapy is associated with around four additional strokes (principally hemorrhagic) and around seven major non-cerebral bleeds per 1000 patients treated. The contraindications for thrombolytic therapy include conditions where there is a significant risk or serious consequences (e.g., coagulation disorders, bleeding disorders, history of cerebral vascular disease, esophageal varices, trauma, hemorrhage, aortic dissection). However, every case should be judged on its merits, as benefits may outweigh the risk of bleeding. Age is not a contraindication. If a patient is allergic to streptokinase or anistreplase, then alteplase or reteplase should be used instead.

The advantages of thrombolytics are that they are cheap, quick, and noninvasive, and the blocked artery is opened in over half cases. The disadvantages are that residual stenosis remains, post-MI ischemia may persist, and systemic and plaque hemorrhages may occur.

Q: What are the indications for primary coronary angioplasty, and how do its results compare with those of thrombolysis?

In primary coronary angioplasty, the patient is brought directly to the cardiac catherization laboratory for coronary angioplasty without the benefit of thrombolysis. Primary coronary angioplasty may be more beneficial than thrombolysis in some, but not all, circumstances. In practice, primary coronary angioplasty is of limited application because the procedure can be carried out only in centers where the necessary staff and equipment are available 24 hours a day. There is still considerable discussion and research going on as to whether primary angioplasty or thrombolytics offer more benefits to the patients. There is a case for primary angioplasty for selected high-risk cases presenting within 12 hours after AMI in a hospital with catheter laboratories. It appears as effective or more effective than thrombolysis, with significantly lower risk of stroke and lower risk of the high mortality associated with cerebral hemorrhage. Some have advocated a policy of thrombolysis followed by angiography in all patients with angioplasty when indicated. Ross et al.[28] found a tPA patency rate of 66% on patients' arrival on the catheter table, which was increased to 77% after intervention. Others believe that at present primary angioplasty cannot be delivered for AMI; therefore, it should be reserved for when lytic therapy has failed. Other advantages of primary coronary angioplasty include residual stenosis that can be cleared and stented, and less post-MI angina and reinfarction. Indications for primary percutaneous transluminal coronary angioplasty (PTCA) are as follows:

1. As an alternative to thrombolytic therapy patients with AMI and ST-segment elevation or new left bundle-branch block (LBBB) who can undergo angioplasty of the infarct-related artery within 12 hours of onset of symptoms or >12 hours if symptoms persist

2. In patients who are within 36 hours of an acute ST elevation/Q wave or new LBBB myocardial infarction who develop cardiogenic shock or are <75 years of age, and revascularization can be performed within 18 hours of onset of shock

3. Patients who have contraindications to thrombolytics

Q: Should beta-blockers, CCBs, ACE inhibitors, and ARBs be prescribed post-MI?

An overall view of randomized controlled trials indicates that both long- and short-term use of beta-blockade in AMI results in major benefits.[21] A meta-analysis of post-MI trials has demonstrated a 23% relative risk reduction in mortality in patients maintained on long-term beta-blocker treatment.[21]

Timolol (initially 5 mg bid, then 10 mg bid), metoprolol (initially 50 mg qds, then 100 mg bid), and propranolol (orally, initially 40 mg qds, then 80 mg bid), all have evidence of long-term cardiac protection following AMI, and they reduce the risk of sudden death, nonfatal reinfarction, and all-cause mortality by 20% to 30%. It is not known if all beta-blockers confer similar protection. Oral beta-blockers should be started within 24 hours of AMI and continued for at least 2 to 3 years. It is not known how long treatment should continue, as the mortality curve diverges after a year, but many patients continue treatment indefinitely, provided there are no troublesome side effects. Patients who have poor left ventricular function or need a diuretic should take a small dose of beta-blocker.

Calcium Channel Blockers (CCBs)

There is no evidence of mortality benefit from these drugs during or after AMI, and there is the risk for increased mortality in people with heart failure. Verapamil may improve outcome when used as an alternative to beta-blocker in patients with good left ventricular function.[29] In MI survivors, rate-limiting calcium antagonists (verapamil[29] and diltiazem[30]) may have prognostic benefit. The advantage is confined to patients without left ventricular impairment. Therefore, verapamil and diltiazem may be options in patients intolerant of beta-blockers. Nifedipine is contraindicated in AMI because of reflex sympathetic activity.

Angiotensin-Converting Enzyme Inhibitors

A number of randomized clinical trials have shown the benefit of using ACE inhibitors early in the course of AMI. ACE inhibitors have been shown to decrease progressive remodeling post-MI and reduce short- and long-term post-MI mortality. The American College of Cardiology (ACC)/American Heart Association (AHA) advocates that all patients should be on ACE inhibitors on hospital discharge unless contraindicated. In post-MI patients with left ventricular dysfunction (LVD), the use of ACE inhibitors reduces the risk of all-cause mortality by 19%, the risk of nonfatal and fatal vascular events (e.g., stroke) by 21%, and the development of severe heart failure by 37% over 42 months' follow-up.[31] ACE inhibitors are useful post-MI, particularly for those with left ventricular dysfunction or when beta-blockers are contraindicated or in high-risk groups with anterior infarcts. The routine use of ACE inhibitors in unselected AMI patients showed some benefit, but those with cardiac failure or ejection fraction of <40% obtained the most gain.[32,33] If ACE inhibitors are initiated in a patient with heart failure with a history of recent MI, within the first week, it significantly reduces mortality and serious cardiovascular events.[34] The Heart Outcomes Prevention Evaluation (HOPE) study now confirms that the use of the ACE inhibitor ramipril, 10 mg/d, reduces the incidence of MI by 22%, stroke by 33%, cardiovascular death by 37%, and the combined primary outcome of these events by 25%. Ramipril also lowered the risk of overt nephropathy by 24%.[4]

Angiotensin Receptor Blockers
The Valsartan in AMI trial demonstrated that ARBs are as effective as ACE inhibitors in reducing the rates of death and other adverse cardiovascular outcomes after MI and should be considered as alternative to ACE inhibitors.[36]

Q: What are the guidelines for cardiac rehabilitation?
The U.S. Agency for Health Care Policy gave the following recommendations: Cardiac rehabilitation should include exercise training, education, counseling, risk reduction, lifestyle modification, and the use of behavioral intervention. The object of cardiac rehabilitation is to improve both the physiological and psychosocial status of the patient. The physiological outcome includes improvement in exercise capacity and exercise habits, and optimization of risk factors, including improvement in blood lipid, weight, blood glucose, blood pressure, and cessation of smoking. Additional goals include enhancement of myocardial perfusion and performance, as well as reduction in the progression of atherosclerosis.[37] The following phases are identified:

Phase I: The inpatient treatment phase. The goal of rehabilitation is to speed recovery and to reduce the risk from the acute phase of MI.
Phase II: The immediate posthospital phase. The patient is at risk of experiencing serious problems such as recurrent myocardial ischemia, heart failure, etc.
Phase III: The specialized skills of physiotherapists, dietitians, cardiac nurses, and clinical psychologists are used to modify lifestyle. The previous advice needs to be reinforced.

Phase IV: Lifelong. The focus is on continuance of a healthy lifestyle and the pursuance of a lifestyle modification program.

Resumption of Normal Physical Activities

There is a tendency to mobilize patients as soon as possible after a heart attack, primarily to prevent thrombosis. Patients are advised to walk while in the hospital, and they should build on this progress when at home. Therefore, the first week at home should be an extension of the last day in the hospital. The patient can climb stairs once a day, but frequent climbing should be avoided. A nap can be taken in the afternoon during the first week at home. Walking should be increased up to 100 meters on a flat surface by the end of the week. Light household work such as washing up or making a cup of tea or a light snack can be undertaken. Hot baths and heavy meals should be avoided.

By the end of the second week, climbing stairs up to four times a day at a gentle pace can be undertaken. Walking distances can be increased up to a quarter of a mile. Walking outdoors on cold and windy days should be avoided. Exercise after a bath or meal should also be avoided.

By the end of the third week stairs can be climbed freely. Daily walks up to half a mile can be undertaken. Household activities can be gradually increased, but lifting objects heavier than 5 kg should be avoided. Heavy household chores such as vacuuming, digging, and cleaning floors may also be too much to do at this stage.

During the fourth week, the walking distance can be increased to 1 mile. Vacuuming, mowing the lawn, etc., can be undertaken.

During fifth and sixth weeks the walking distance should be increased to 1 to 2 miles, and this could include small hills. Other daily activities should be gradually increased.

Resumption of Working and Driving

Patients can return to work as soon as they feel physically and psychologically capable of doing so. Following a heart attack, a patient who is symptom- and complication-free can be expected to return to work in 4 to 6 weeks. A car should not be driven for at least 1 month following a heart attack or a heart operation, provided recovery has been uncomplicated, and the doctor's approval has been sought.

Resumption of Sexual Intercourse

There are no fixed rules. Sexual activity can be started when one feels up to it. Having sexual intercourse does not put an extra strain on the heart. The maximal heart rate with sexual activity is approximately 120 beats per minute (less if the patient is taking rate-limiting drugs such as a beta-blocker) and this will last for less than 3 minutes. The energy demand or metabolic equivalent of intercourse varies from 2 to 6 METs depending on how vigorous it is. This energy demand and the oxygen cost to the heart are similar to climbing two flights of stairs or performing ordinary occupational tasks.

After a heart attack, the patient may have sexual intercourse after 2 weeks, provided there are no complications. After a heart operation, the patient may resume sexual activity when he or she feels up to it. After angioplasty sexual activity can be resumed within a few days. If angina develops during sexual intercourse, glycerine trinitrate spray sublingually may be taken. Those who get breathless may find that their partner should assume a more active role, such as taking the superior position during sexual intercourse. Sexual activity should be avoided for 2 hours after a meal or a hot bath.

Secondary Prevention

The following measures are essential:

- Lifestyle measures, which include dietary (TLC or Mediterranean diet), smoking cessation, increased physical activity, weight maintenance (BMI 18.5–24.9 kg/m^2, waist circumference in men <40 in [102 cm], in women <35 in [88 cm]), targeting BP (<140/90 mm Hg, <130/80 mm Hg if chronic renal failure or diabetes), and blood glucose to required levels (HA$_{1c}$ <7%).
- Aspirin 75–160 mg daily. If intolerant to aspirin, clopidogrel 75 mg daily should be taken; combination of two should be considered. In case of true aspirin allergy, warfarin therapy with a target international normalized ratio (INR) of 2.5 to 3.5 is a useful alternative to clopidogrel in post-MI patients less than 75 years of age who are at low risk of bleeding.
- Post-MI beta-blocker. If contraindicated, use rate-limiting CCBs (i.e., verapamil and diltiazem).
- Lipid-lowering drugs, usually statin; LDL-C goal <100 mg/dl (2.6 mmol/L), treat elevated triglyceride or low HDL as previously discussed.
- ACE inhibitor, particularly those who have LVD or diabetes. Start early in high-risk patients and continue indefinitely. If intolerant, then ARBs should be given.
- Long-term aldosterone blockade is indicated in patients without significant renal dysfunction or hyperkalemia who are already

receiving ACE inhibitors, have left ventricular ejection fraction ≤40%, or have either heart failure or diabetes.[19]

- Treadmill exercise testing should assess all patients on discharge, as those not assessed or who have contraindication are at four-fold risk of mortality.[38] The presence of ST-segment changes on ECG, abnormal blood pressure response, and angina at a sub-maximum level before hospital discharge or 1 month after AMI predicts the risk of ischemic events, the need for a revascular-ization procedure, and overall increased cardiac mortality. Evi-dence of ischemia at low exercise indicates multivessel disease or unresolved coronary flow limitation. Some of these patients may need further investigations.

- Before the patient is discharged from the hospital, the patient and relatives are given sufficient information and training to deal with impending long-term complications.

- Patient should undergo psychological evaluation regarding depression, anxiety, and insomnia.

Q: Does blood sugar affect prognosis post-MI?

A diabetic patient who suffers AMI has a long-term mortality nearly twice that of a nondiabetic.[39] Up to 10% of patients admitted with AMI suffer undiagnosed diabetes. Patients on admission with blood sugar <7 mmol/L (125 mg/dL) usually have an uncomplicated outcome, while those with blood sugar >9 mmol/L (165 mg/dL) are more likely to develop complications. Increased mortality in dia-betes is related to cardiac failure, the size of the coronary afflic-tion, and the specific diabetic cardiomyopathy. The combination of low insulin and increased fatty acids (result of catecholamine release) increases myocardial oxygen demand. Therefore, control-ling blood glucose and fatty acid with IV insulin infusion prevents myocardial deterioration and reduces mortality and morbidity.[40] Postmyocardial treatment with beta-blockers, ACE inhibitors, and statins reduces mortality in diabetics.

Q: What are the detrimental effects of myocardial remodeling, and how can they be reduced?

During the early stages of AMI, infarct expansion may occur in which the affected ventricular area enlarges, which represents thin-ning and dilatation of the necrotic zone of the tissue. As a result the ventricular size increases, but this has adverse effect as it (1) increases wall stress, (2) impairs ventricular contractibility, and (3) increases the chances of aneurysm formation. In addition to infarct expansion, the adjoining noninfarcted area also dilates, due to increased wall stress. This process is initiated during the early post-MI period, but continues over the next few weeks or months. In the beginning, the initial dilatation helps to increase cardiac output, but ultimately it predisposes to heart failure and ventricular arrhythmias. Ventricular remodeling is detrimental, and can be modified by certain interventions, such as ACE inhibitors.

References

1. Braunwald E. Application of Current Guidelines to the Management of Unstable Angina Non-ST-Elevation Myocardial Infarction. Circulation 2003;108:III28–37.
2. Stevenson R, Wilkinson P, Merchant B. Relative value of clinical variables, treadmill stress testing and Holter ST monitoring for post infarction risk stratification. Am J Cardiol 1994;70:233–240.
3. Galvani M, Ottani F, Oltrona L, et al. NT-proBNP on admission has prognostic value across the whole spectrum of ACS. Circulation 2004;110:128–134.
4. Antman EM, Cohen M, Bernink PJLM, et al. The TIMI Risk Score for Unstable Angina/Non-ST Elevation MI. JAMA 2000;284:835–842.
5. CAPRIE Steering Committee. A randomised double blind trial of clopidogrel versus aspirin in patients at risk of ischaemic events. Lancet 1996;348:1329–1339.
6. RISC Study. Risk of MI and death during treatment with low dose aspirin and IV heparin in men with unstable coronary artery disease. Lancet 1990;336:826–830.
7. Anti-platelet Trialists' Collaboration. Overview 1: Prevention of death, myocardial infarction and stroke by prolonged anti-platelet therapy in various categories of patients. BMJ 1994;308:81–106.
8. CURE Investigation. Effects of clopidogrel in addition to aspirin in patients with acute coronary syndromes without ST-segment elevation. N Engl J Med 2001;345:494–502.
9. King DF, Califf RM, Millar DP, et al. Clinical outcome of therapeutic agents that block the glycoprotein IIb/IIIa integrin in ischemic heart disease. Circulation 1998;98:2829–2835.
10. Brauwald E, Antman E, Beasley J, et al. ACC/AHA guidelines update for the management of patients with unstable angina and non-ST-segment elevation myocardial infarction. Circulation 2002;106:1893.
11. Oler A, Whooley MA, Oler J, et al. Adding heparin to aspirin reduces the incidence of myocardial infarction and death in patients with unstable angina. A meta-analysis. JAMA 1996;276:811–815.
12. Antman EM, McAbe CH, Gurfinkel EP, et al. Enoxaparin prevents death cardiac ischemic events in unstable angina/non-Q-wave myocardial infarction. Results of thrombolysis in myocardial infarction (TIMI) IIB trial. Circulation 1999;100:1593–1601.

13. Schwartz GG, Olsson AG, Ezekowitz MD, et al., for the Myocardial Ischemia Reduction with Aggressive Cholesterol Lowering (MIRACL) Study Investigators. Effects of atorvastatin on early recurrent ischemic events in acute coronary syndromes: the MIRACL study a randomised controlled trial. JAMA 2001;285:1711–1718.

14. Mair J, Morandell D, Genser N, et al. Equivalent early sensitivities of myoglobin, creatine kinase MB mass, creatine kinase isoform ratio and cardiac troponin l and T for acute myocardial infarction. Clin Chem 1995;41:1266–1272.

15. Mair J. Progress in myocardial damage detection: new biochemical markers for clinicians. Crit Rev Lab Sci 1997;34:1–66.

16. Herren R, Mackway-Jones K, Richards R, et al. Diagnostic cohort study of an emergency department-based 6-hour rule-out protocol for myocardial damage. Br Med J 2001;323:1–4.

17. Gibson RS. Non Q wave myocardial infarction, prognosis and management. Curr Prob Cardiol 1988;13(2):8–72.

18. ISIS-1. Randomised trial of intravenous Atenolol among 16,027 cases of acute myocardial infarction: First International Study of Infarct Survival Collaborative Group. Lancet 1986;2:57–66.

19. Antman EM, Anbe DT, Armstrong PW, et al. ACC/AHA guidelines for the management of patients with ST-elevation myocardial infarction. Executive summary. Circulation 2004;110:588–656.

20. ISIS-2. Randomised trial of intravenous streptokinase, oral aspirin, both or neither among 17,187 cases of suspected acute myocardial infarction. Second International Study of Infarct Survival collaborative Group. Lancet 1988;2:349–360.

21. Freemantle N, Cleland J, Young P, Mason J, Harrison J. Beta-blockade after myocardial infarction: systemic review and meta regression analysis. BMJ 1999;318:1730–1737.

22. Jafri SM, Gheorghiade M, Goldstein S. Oral anticoagulants for secondary prevention after myocardial infarction with special reference to the Warfarin Reinfarction Study (WARIS). Prog Cardiovasc Dis 1992; 34:317–324.

23. ASPECT Research Group. Effect of long-term oral anticoagulant treatment on mortality and cardiovascular mortality after MI. Lancet 1994; 343:499–503.

24. Malmberg K, Ryden L, Efendic S, et al., for the diabetes Mellitus, Insulin Glucose Infusion in Acute Myocardial Infarction (DIGAMI) Study Group. Randomized trial of insulin-glucose infusion followed by subcutaneous insulin treatment in diabetic patients with acute myocardial infarction: effect on mortality at one year. J Am Coll Cardiol 1995; 26:57–65.

25. GISS-2. A factorial randomised trial of alteplase vs. streptokinase and heparin vs. no heparin among 12,490 patients with acute myocardial infarction. Lancet 1990;336:65–71.

26. ISIS-3. A randomised comparison of streptokinase vs. tissue plasminogen activator vs. anistreplase and of aspirin plus heparin vs. aspirin alone 41,299 cases of suspected myocardial infarction. Third

International Study of Infarct Survival Collaborative Group. Lancet 1992;339:753–770.

27. The GUSTO Investigators. An international randomised trial comparing four thrombolytic strategies for acute myocardial infarction. N Engl J Med 1993;329:673–682.

28. Ross AM, Coyne KS, Reiner JS, et al. A randomised trial comparing primary angioplasty with a strategy of short-acting thrombolysis and immediate planned rescue angioplasty in an acute myocardial infarction: the PACT Trial. PACT Investigators. Plasminogen Activator Angioplasty Compatibility Trial. J Am Coll Cardiol 1999;34:1954–1962.

29. The Danish Study Group on Verapamil in Myocardial Infarction. Effect of verapamil on mortality and major events after acute myocardial infarction (The Danish Verapamil Infarction Trial-DAVITT II). Am J Cardiol 1990;79:779–785.

30. The Multicenter Diltiazem Post Infarction Trial (MDPITT) research group. The effects of diltiazem on mortality and reinfarction after myocardial infarction. N Engl J Med 1988;319:385–392.

31. Pfeller MA, Braunwald E, Moyle LA, et al. Effects of captopril on mortality and morbidity in patients with left ventricular dysfunction after myocardial infarction: results of the survival and ventricular enlargement trial (SAVE). N Engl J Med 1992;327:669–677.

32. GISS-3. Effects of lisinopril and transdermal glyceryl trinitrate singly and together on 6-week mortality and ventricular function after acute myocardial infarction. Lancet 1994;343:1115–1122.

33. ISIS-4. A randomized trial comparing oral captopril versus placebo, oral mononitrate vs. placebo, and intravenous magnesium sulphate vs. control among 58,043 patients with suspected acute myocardial infarction. Lancet 1995;345:669–685.

34. Sutton MS. Should ACE inhibitors to be used routinely after infarction? Perspectives from the SAVE trial. Br Heart J 1994;71:115–118.

35. HOPE study. Effects of ramopril on CV and microvascular outcomes in people with diabetes mellitus. Lancet 2000;355:253–259.

36. Pfeffer MA, Mc Murray JJV, Velazques EJ, et al., for Valsartan in AMI investigators. Valsartan, captopril, or both in MI complicated by heart failure, left ventricular dysfunction, or both. N Engl J Med 2003; 349:1893–1906.

37. Wenger NK, Froelicher ES, Smith LK, et al. Cardiac rehabilitation. Clinical Practice Guideline No. 17. AHCRP Publication No. 96-0672. Rockville, MD: US Department of Health and Human Services, Public Health Service, Agency for Health Care Policy and Research and the National Heart, Lung, and Blood Institute, 1975.

38. Villella M, Villella A, Barlera S, Franzosi MG, Maggiono AP. Prognostic significance of double product and inadequate double product response to maximum symptom-limited exercise stress testing after myocardial infarction in 6296 patients treated with thrombolytic agents. GISSI-2 Investigators. Groppo Italiano per Lo Studio della Sopravvivenza nell-Infarto Miocardico. Am Heart J 1999;137:443–452.

39. Mak KH, Moliterno DJ, Granger CB, et al. Influence of diabetes mellitus on clinical outcome in the thrombolytic era of acute myocardial infarction. J Am Coll Cardiol 1997;30:171–179.
40. Malmberg K, for the DIGAMI Study Group. Prospective randomised study of intensive insulin treatment on long-term survival after acute myocardial infarction in patients with diabetes mellitus. BMJ 1997;314: 1512–1515.

Chapter 9
Heart Failure

It has been estimated that heart failure affects more than 4 million patients in the United States and that more than 500,000 people are diagnosed with new heart failure each year.[1] In the Studies of Left Ventricular Dysfunction (SOLVD)[2] coronary artery disease accounted for almost 75% of the cases of chronic heart failure in white male patients, although in the Framingham heart study, coronary heart disease accounted for only 46% of cases of heart failure in men and 27% of chronic heart failure cases in women. Coronary artery disease and hypertension (either alone or in combination) were implicated as the cause in over 90% of cases of heart failure in the Framingham study (Table 9.1).

Q: What is the pathophysiology of congestive heart failure?
Congestive heart failure (CHF) is a clinical syndrome of breathlessness, effort intolerance, and edema caused by a variety of cardiac abnormalities. These abnormalities include, rhythm problems (e.g., atrial fibrillation), heart valve disease, and, most commonly, left ventricular systolic dysfunction (LVSD). With the advent of new investigative procedures, it has now become easier to diagnose heart failure early, and this enables early institution of treatment.

PATHOPHYSIOLOGY
Heart failure is a condition in which the heart fails to discharge its contents adequately. It is associated with abnormalities of cardiac function, skeletal muscle, and renal function; stimulation of sympathetic nervous system; and a complex pattern of neurohormonal changes. Except in cases of valvular heart failure, the primary abnormality is the impairment of left ventricular function. Reduced cardiac output causes activation of several neurohormonal compensatory mechanisms. Stimulation of sympathetic system leads to tachycardia, increased myocardial contractility, and peripheral vasoconstriction. Activation of the renin-angiotensin-aldosterone

TABLE 9.1. New York Heart Association (NYHA) classification of heart failure

Grade	Criteria
I	Symptoms only occur on severe exertion; an almost normal lifestyle is possible
II	Symptoms on moderate exertion; patient has to avoid certain situations (i.e., carrying shopping bags, climbing several stairs)
III	Symptoms occur on mild exertion
IV	Symptoms occur frequently, even at rest

system also leads to vasoconstriction (due to angiotensin) and an increase in blood volume, with retention of salt and water (due to aldosterone). Blood concentration of vasopressin and natriuretic peptide increases. There is also increasing cardiac dilatation. There are three natriuretic peptides. Atrial natriuretic peptide (ANP) is released from the atria in response to stretch, leading to natriuresis and vasodilatation. Brain natriuretic peptide (BNP) is also released from the heart, predominantly from the ventricles. ANP and BNP have similar action. C-type natriuretic peptide is limited to the vascular endothelium and central nervous system and has only limited effects on natriuresis and vasodilatation.

Myocardial Remodeling, Hibernation, and Stunning
Following heart attack, cardiac contractility is often impaired, and neurohormonal activation causes regional eccentric and concentric hypertrophy of the noninfarcted segment with expansion of the infarcted zone. This is known as remodeling. Myocardial dysfunction may also occur in response to "stunning" (postischemic dysfunction), which describes the delayed recovery of myocardial function despite the restoration of coronary artery flow, in the absence of irreversible damage. This is in contrast to "hibernating" myocardium, which describes persistent myocardial dysfunction at rest, secondary to reduced myocardial perfusion, although cardiac myocytes remain viable and myocardial contraction may improve with revascularization.

Some patients may develop heart failure as a result of diastolic dysfunction.

MANAGEMENT

Q: What investigations should be done in the diagnosis of heart failure?

The following investigations are usually recommended:

- Echocardiography is the most important technique used in the diagnosis of heart failure even in the presymptomatic stages. Two-dimensional Doppler echocardiography allows quantification of global and regional left and right ventricular systolic function. An ejection fraction of <45%, with or without symptoms, may be accepted as evidence of left ventricular dysfunction. Echocardiography can also exclude other causes of heart failure, such as mitral stenosis, mitral regurgitation, aortic valve disease, pericardial disease, restrictive (in some cases), and hypertrophic cardiomyopathies.
- Recently, the facility has become available to test blood level of BNP, thus enabling diagnosis of heart failure with single blood test.
- Chest x-ray and electrocardiogram.
- Blood tests for anemia, liver function test, urea, and electrolytes.

Further Techniques

Radionuclide Ventriculography and Angiography

In a minority of cases cardiac catheterization is necessary to determine the cause of heart failure, including valvular and ischemic etiologies. These methods measure left ventricular size and function. Some techniques can also make it possible to analyze diastolic filling and right ventricular function. Images may be obtained in patients in whom echocardiography is not possible. The most common method labels red cells with technetium-99m and acquires 16 or 32 frames per heartbeat by synchronizing ("gating") imaging with echocardiography. This allows the assessment of ejection fraction, systolic filling rate, diastolic emptying rate, and wall motion abnormalities. These variables can be assessed, if necessary, during rest and exercise; this method is ideal for the serial reassessment of ejection fraction. Angiography should be considered in those who suffer recurrent ischemic chest pain.

Ambulatory 24-Hour Electrocardiogram (ECG) Monitoring

This monitoring detects asymptomatic ventricular arrhythmia, which is common in patients with heart failure.

Exercise Treadmill Stress Testing (EST)

Treadmill stress testing is used to classify the severity of heart failure, to assess progress, and to evaluate the effectiveness of treatment. When combined with measurements of gas exchange during prolonged exercise assessment, exercise stress testing can provide a useful quantitative index of functional capacity.

Pulmonary Function Tests

These tests exclude pulmonary causes of breathlessness.

Q: What are the current strategies in the treatment of congestive heart failure?

Recent studies show that angiotensin-converting enzyme (ACE) inhibitors, the aldosterone antagonists (e.g., spironolactone), and beta-blockers improve symptoms, delay symptomatic deterioration, greatly reduce the need for hospital admission, and substantially improve survival. Women of childbearing age with advanced heart failure should use a reliable contraceptive method due to the risk of high mortality and morbidity during pregnancy and delivery. Lifestyle issues (e.g., smoking, excessive alcohol intake) need to be addressed. Regular exercise should be advised. Vaccinations with influenza and pneumococcal vaccine should be encouraged. Patients should avoid foods rich in salt. Fluid intake should be restricted to 1.5–2 L daily in those with advanced heart failure and requiring high dose of diuretics. Patients should be advised that if they gain weight suddenly, they should seek medical attention.

Current Strategies

The standard treatment of chronic heart failure with left ventricular systolic dysfunction includes ACE inhibitors, diuretics, and beta-blockers. The general sequence is to start with ACE inhibitors as well as diuretics. If the patient does not tolerate ACE inhibitors, then angiotensin receptor blockers (ARBs) (or hydralazine plus isosorbide dinitrate) may be substituted.

For patients without recent clinical deterioration or volume overload, a beta-blocker should be added. Digoxin should be added if the symptom persists. In class IV heart failure, spironolactone may be tried. At this stage direct-current (DC) shock may be considered for atrial fibrillation. An implantable defibrillator should be considered in sustained ventricular arrhythmia.

In those with mild evidence of salt retention, nonloop diuretics (e.g., hydrochlorothiazide 12.5 to 25 mg daily) may be sufficient. However, most patients with symptomatic heart failure need a loop diuretic (e.g., furosemide 20 to 40 mg daily, or bumetamide 1 to 10 mg daily). In the usual practice, the patient may be started on furosemide 40 mg daily. A combinaion of loop diuretics and thiazides may be effective in resistant cases. If the patient gains 1 to 3 kg of weight due to excess fluid retention, a nonloop diuretic such as metolazole 2.5 to 5 mg daily may be given, half an hour to 1 hour before taking a loop diuretic. Metolazole exerts an effect on the proximal tubule, causing increased delivery of sodium chloride to the loop of Henle, thereby facilitating the action of the loop diuretic. Once a patient achieves a baseline weight, metolazole is stopped. Serum potassium should be monitored while a patient is taking an ACE inhibitor or diuretic because hyper- and hypokalemia can precipitate ventricular arrhythmias.

Diuretics

Diuretics remain the first-line treatment.

Thiazide diuretics act within 1 to 2 hours after the oral dose, and the duration of action lasts from 12 to 24 hours; therefore, they should be taken in the early morning. Chlortalidone (chlorthalidone), a thiazide-related drug, has a longer duration of action than thiazide and may be given on alternate days.

Loop diuretics inhibit reabsorption of sodium from the ascending loop of Henle in the renal tubule and are powerful diuretics. Furosemide (40 mg) and bumetanide (1 mg) are similar in potency. Their effect starts in 1 hour, and the duration of action is 6 hours. Their side effects include hypokalemia, hyponatremia, rashes, and disturbance of blood lipids and sugar levels.

The distal tubular diuretics (spironolactone, triamterene, and amiloride) do not lose potassium or raise uric acid and blood sugar. Triamterene and amiloride retain potassium. The Randomized Aldactone Evaluation Study (RALES) showed that spironolactone significantly reduced morbidity and mortality in patients with moderate or severe heart failure.[3] It is used in a low dose of 25 mg daily in heart failure. Potassium-sparing diuretics are not used alone but in combination with a potassium-depleting one.

Angiotensin-Converting Enzyme (ACE) Inhibitors

The Studies of Left Ventricular Dysfunction (SOLVD) trial has firmly established the role of ACE inhibitors as the mainstay of treatment in heart failure, but diuretics remain important as co-therapy in symptomatic patients.[2] More recently, clinical trial evidence has supported a role of ACE inhibitors in preventing progression of heart failure in post–myocardial infarction (MI). Angiotensin-converting enzyme inhibitors improve symptoms and quality of life, increase exercise tolerance, and reduce mortality and morbidity.

Angiotensin-converting enzyme inhibitors should be prescribed in all cases of congestive heart failure due to left ventricular dysfunction even if a patient has responded to diuretics. Larger doses of ACE inhibitors are more effective (e.g., enalapril 10 to 20 mg bid, captopril 50 mg tid, lisinopril 30 mg daily, and perindropril 4 mg daily). ACE inhibitors reduce both preload and afterload, enhancing ventricular emptying. They may have other additional modes of action. A combination of a diuretic and an ACE inhibitor has many advantages. In moderate to severe heart failure ACE inhibitors can show substantial clinical benefit. Diuretics should be withheld for 24 hours before the ACE inhibitor can be initiated. Initially a small dosage is given at bedtime to avoid postural hypotension. Some patients may need to be hospitalized if they need ACE inhibitors and are already taking a diuretic. If a patient is not taking a diuretic, then an ACE inhibitor can be started without delay and diuretics can be added when necessary without waiting. There is evidence that although ACE inhibitors may be beneficial when prescribed alone in patients with a symptomatic left ventricular dysfunction, they should be given in conjunction with a diuretic in patients with symptomatic heart failure.

Angiotensin Receptor Blockers

The angiotensin receptor blockers (ARBs) have a great advantage in not causing cough, and there is evidence from studies that they (particularly losartan, valsartan and candersartan)[5] are an appropriate alternative in patients who develop intolerable side effects from ACE inhibitors. The Evaluation of Losartan in the Elderly Study, which compared losartan with captopril in patients aged 65 or over with mild to severe congestive heart failure did not confirm that losartan was superior to captopril.[4] (ARBs are described in Chapter 4.)

Beta-Blockers

Beta-blockers have traditionally been contraindicated in heart failure. But now there is enough evidence to support the use of beta-blockers in patients with chronic stable heart failure resulting from left ventricular dysfunction. The use of beta-blockers with conventional treatment (with diuretics) and ACE inhibitors results in improvement in left ventricular function, and survival, as well as a reduction in hospital admissions. Beta-blockers should be prescribed for all stable patients with CHF, and the dose at which they are started should be very low (e.g., initial doses are carvedilol

3.125 mg [target 25 mg bid], bisoprolol 1.25 mg [target 10 mg daily], and metoprolol CR/XL 12.5 to 25 mg [target 50 mg] daily) and titrated slowly over a period of weeks or months. Initially, some symptomatic deterioration may occur but it usually resolves with adjustment of the diuretic dose. Any dose of BB is better than none. Even in class IV heart failure BB should be tried but only in hospitalized patient. In the United Kingdom, carvedilol is licensed for mild to moderate symptoms and bisoprolol for moderate to severe heart failure.

The Cardiac Insufficiency Bisoprolol Study II (CIBIS-II), which included patients with New York Heart Association (NYHA) classes III and IV, was stopped prematurely after it was found that the bisoprolol-treated group had a highly significantly better survival rate than the placebo group.[6] The Metroprolol CR/XL Randomized Intervention Trial in Congestive Heart Failure showed that metoprolol provided a 34% relative risk reduction in mortality and a 41% relative risk reduction in sudden death in patients with class II to class IV heart failure.[7] These figures are similar to those of CIBIS-II. The respective risk reductions with bisoprolol were 34% for total mortality and 44% for sudden death. Carvedilol Prospective Randomized Cumulative Survival Study (COPERNICUS) showed benefit of carvediol even in patients of severe heart failure.[8]

Vasodilators

Vasodilators reduce cardiac workload by causing venous dilatation. Nitrates and hydralazine are commonly used. Nitrates are a useful addition to the therapeutic options for heart failure, but the ACE inhibitors have largely supplanted them. In general, oral nitrates should be considered in patients with angina and impaired left ventricular systolic function. The combination of nitrates and hydralazine is an alternative regimen in patients with severe renal impairment, in whom ACE inhibitors and angiotensin II receptor antagonists are contraindicated. Hydralazine is given initially in the dosage of 25 mg tid.

Digoxin

The Digitalis Investigation Group (DIG) studied over 7500 patients with heart failure, and found no significant effect of digoxin on mortality, but there was a reduction in the hospitalization rate in the digoxin group as compared to placebo.[6] The DIG trial confirms that there are no long-term safety concerns when digitalis is used to improve exercise tolerance and quality of life. It also reduces hospitalization due to worsening heart failure. Symptomatic patients with preserved left ventricular function derive benefits similar to those experienced by patients with poor systolic function.

Some physicians question the use of digoxin in patients with sinus rhythm, but its use in atrial fibrillation remains undisputed. Digoxin also improves symptoms in patients with CHF due to LVSD and who are in sinus rhythm. Digoxin is probably more useful, in those who remain symptomatic despite the use of ACE inhibitors, diuretics, and beta-blockers, in those who have cardiomegaly on chest x-ray, and in those who have poor left ventricular function. Blood levels of digoxin help to exclude toxicity and to ensure a therapeutic level, but have no relation with its efficacy. The dose of digoxin is 0.125–0.25 mg/d or 0.125 mg alternate days in elderly.

Nonglycoside Inotropic Agents

These sympathomimetic agents (e.g., dobutamine and dopexamine) are given intravenously and are useful for short periods in the treatment of heart failure. Their use is limited, as they are not available in oral forms. Studies also have not supported improved survival with their use.

Calcium Channel Blockers

Most calcium channel blockers are contraindicated in heart failure. If there is coexistent angina, then either amlodipine or felodipine should be used. Long-acting dihydropyridine calcium channel blockers generally have a neutral effect in heart failure.

Antithrombotic Treatment

The combination of atrial fibrillation and heart failure (or evidence of left ventricular dysfunction on echocardiography) is associated with increased risk of thromboembolism, which is reduced by the long-term use of warfarin. Aspirin alone is not suitable for this purpose.

Acute Heart Failure

For the treatment of acute heart failure, the following options should be considered:

- Sit the patient upright.
- Administer a high concentration of oxygen via a face mask.
- Assess fluid balance.
- Estimate blood gases.
- Prescribe IV loop diuretics.
- Prescribe parenteral opiates as an adjunct to relieve anxiety and pain.
- Prescribe nitrates.
- Prescribe inotropic agents (e.g., dobutamine and dopamine) in resistant cases.

References

1. Hunt SA, Baker DW, Chin MH, et al. ACC/AHA guidelines for the evaluation and management of chronic heart failure in the adult. Circulation 2001;104:2996–3007.

2. The Studies of Left Ventricular Dysfunction (SOLVD) investigators. Effects on enalapril on survival in patients with reduced left ventricular ejection fraction and congestive heart failure. N Engl J Med 1991;325: 293–303.

3. Pitt B, Zannad F, Remme WJ, et al. The Randomized Aldactone Evaluation Study (RALES) investigator. The effect of spironolactone on morbidity and mortality in patients with severe heart failure. N Engl J Med 1999;341:709–717.

4. Pitt B, Pool-Wilson PA, Segal R, et al. The ELITE II investigators. Effect of losartan compared with captopril on mortality in patients with symptomatic heart failure: randomized trial – the Losartan Heart Failure Survival Study ELITE II. Lancet. 2000;355:1582–1587.

5. Young JB, Dunlap ME, Pfeffer A, et al. for the candesartan in heart failure assessment in mortality and morbidity (CHARM) investigators and Committees. Mortality and morbidity reduction with candesartan in patients with chronic heart failure and left ventricular systolic dysfunction: Results of the CHARM low-left ventricular ejection fraction trials. Circulation 2004;110:2618–2626.

6. The Cardiac Insufficiency Bisoprolol Study II (CIBIS-II): a randomized trial. Lancet 1999;353:9–13.

7. The MERIT-HF Study Group (Deedwania, Gottlieb S, Principal Investigators, USA). Effect of metoprolol CR/XL in chronic heart failure: Metoprolol CR/XL randomized intervention trial in congestive heart failure. Lancet 1999;353:2001–2007.

8. Packer M, Coats AJ, Fowler MB, et al. Effect of carvedilol on survival in severe chronic heart failure. N Engl J Med 2001 May 31;344(22): 1651–1658.

9. The Digitalis Investigation Group. The effect of digoxin on mortality and morbidity in patients with heart failure. N Engl J Med 1997;336:525–533.

Chapter 10
Arrhythmias

Q: What is the mechanism of production of arrhythmias?
The way the arrhythmias are produced is fairly well understood. There are two major mechanisms: reentry and altered automaticity. In a reentrant arrhythmia a wave of electrical activity circulates in a so-called circuit movement. The circuit size can vary from less than a millimeter to one involving almost whole myocardium. Very small circuits are termed microreentry, and large circuits are macroreentry. In the second important mechanism, called altered automaticity, a cell or cells become pacemakers. They override the heart's normal pacemaker (sinus node), and produce an ectopic rhythm.

Reentrant arrhythmias involve abnormal pathways and routes of conduction. These may either be created by disease, such as myocardial infarction (MI) or Wolff-Parkinson-White syndrome. Arrhythmias due to abnormal automaticity usually arise in damaged tissues, for example, in myocardial damage caused by myocardial ischemia, or in tissues subjected to abnormal conditions, such as the atria in mitral stenosis.

Myocardial infarction may lead to various types of arrhythmias, depending largely on the size of an infarct, extent of functional loss of myocardium, and the severity and extent of coronary heart disease. Abnormal electrical activity in myocardium damaged by ischemia/infarction can lead to dysrhythmias. Important contributory factors include electrolyte imbalance (e.g., raised potassium), hypoxia, acidosis, and release of catecholamines and free radicals after myocardial ischemia.

Many patients have increased activity of the autonomic nervous system as a result of pain, anxiety, and fear. Sympathetic overactivity occurs in over 50% of MI sufferers, particularly with anterior MI. Approximately, 15% suffer from atrial fibrillation and 20% have extremely serious dysrhythmias. About 30% of patients have slow rhythm especially in inferior MI. It is important to look at the issues surrounding arrhythmias caused by coronary heart disease

(CHD). Myocardial ischemia causes biochemical alteration, whereas MI creates areas of electrical inactivity with block conduction, which lead to arrhythmias. Arrhythmia arising during the first 24 hours of onset of MI is not prognostic, unlike the ones arising after 24 hours.

Q: What are the important supraventricular arrhythmias?

Supraventricular tachyarrhythmia (SVT) arises due to excitation occurring in either the atria or atrioventricular node (hence termed supraventricular). The heart beats at the rate of 140 to 220 beats per minute. If not treated, the attack may last from a few seconds to a few hours. During an attack, the patient may feel faint or breathless or may pass urine more frequently. Excessive intake of tea, coffee, or alcohol may precipitate the attack. Tachycardia may come in attacks (paroxysmal supraventricular tachycardia [PSVT]) and stops spontaneously. The most common forms of PSVT are atrioventricular nodal reentrant tachycardia, atrio-ventricular reciprocating, and atrial tachycardia:

ATRIAL FIBRILLATION

Q: What are the causes of atrial fibrillation and how should it be managed?

Atrial fibrillation (AF) is the most common arrhythmia, occurring in 0.3% to 0.4% of the general population and increasing with age. The incidence of atrial tachyarrhythmia during preinfarction is about 10% to 20%. The incidence of AF after acute MI (AMI) has been reduced since the advent of thrombolysis, but is still indicative of a poor prognosis.[1] Atrial fibrillation has an irregular rhythm of 350 to 600 beats per minute, but with a block it reduces to about 160 beats per minute. P waves are not identifiable. Atrial fibrillation occurs within 72 hours of the onset of AMI. It is associated with long-term mortality, reinfarction, ventricular arrhythmias, and cardiogenic shock. A wide variety of conditions can lead to atrial fibrillation. In Western countries, coronary artery disease and hypertension account for more than 60% of cases. Rheumatic mitral disease may be cause of atrial fibrillation in developing countries. Other frequent causes include cardiomyopathy, thyrotoxicosis, congenital heart disease, and sick-sinus syndrome. Atrial fibrillation is present in about 15% of patients with untreated thyrotoxic patients, and is associated with the so-called holiday heart syndrome that is due to excessive alcohol intake. In up to 10% of cases, no cause can be detected, and they are termed "lone" or idiopathic atrial fibrillation.

Patients may present with palpation, breathlessness, chest pain, or dizziness. In some, particularly in the elderly, AF may be an incidental finding. The most important complication of AF is thromboembolism, leading to stroke or transient ischemic attack (TIA). The aim of treatment in AF is controlling the rapid heart rate and irregular rhythm and preventing thrombus formation by the use of aspirin or warfarin. The regular rhythm can be restored by electric shock or by the use of drugs, such as amiodarone ibutilide, procainamide, flecanide and propaffnone.[2] Controlling the rate is more important than reverting to normal. Heart rate can be controlled with digoxin, diltiazem, verapamil, and beta-blockers. If these fail, or the symptoms are severe, then amiodarone or dofetilide (not available in the U.K.) is indicated. Dofetilide is quite successful in treating AF caused by MI with left ventricular dysfunction, but continuous electrocardiogram (ECG) monitoring is recommended while administering this drug. Elective cardioversion should be considered if required. All patients are anticoagulated with warfarin. If there is a contraindication for the use of warfarin, then aspirin 75 mg daily could be used. Clinical trials, however, show that warfarin reduces the risk of stroke by 60% while aspirin does so by 20%. If medical therapy fails, radiofrequency catheter ablation of AV node may be considered.

Atrial flutter is characterized by rapid atrial activity at the rate of 180 to 350 beats per minute and occurs in patients with preexisting heart disease. With block the ventricular rate reduces to about 150 beats per minute. The treatment of choice includes electric cardioversion or temporary/permanent pacemaker. For patients who have no immediate need for DC shock, drugs similar to those used for atrial fibrillation may be tried. Radiofrequency catheter ablation is often a better alternative to drug treatment.

Q: What are the different types of atrioventricular block?

Defective conduction through the conductive system can lead to heart block. Myocardial ischemia can cause a variety of conduction disturbances involving both the atrioventricular node and infranodal focus. Although atrioventricular (AV) block or bundle-branch block carries an independent risk for mortality and inpatient complications, the use of pacing during this period does not alter mortality. First-degree heart block, like complete heart block, occurs more often with inferior MI, whereas second-degree heart block and conduction disturbances involving the left and right bundle branches occur more often in anterior MI. There are three types of heart blocks: First-degree heart block is the most common conduction defect, occurring in about 14% of MI cases. It is seen in ECG as prolongation of the PR interval (>0.2 sec/>5 small squares). The relation between P waves and the QRS complex, however, remains normal. First-degree heart block is usually benign and does not require any treatment.

Second-degree heart block is characterized by intermittent failure of AV conduction; as a result P waves are not always followed by QRS complex. There are two types:

1. Mobitz type I (Wenckebach type), in which the PR interval progressively increases until a beat is dropped. It is practically always due to impaired conduction and is benign.

2. Mobitz type II, characterized by sudden and unpredictable loss of AV conduction, without preceding gradual lengthening of the PR interval. This type is usually due to bundle block beyond the AV node, resulting in wide QRS complexes, like those of right and left bundle-branch block. Unlike type I, this type usually requires pacemaker, even in asymptomatic patients.

Third-degree heart blocks (complete heart block) entails complete failure of conduction between the atria and ventricle. MI is the most common cause, and a permanent pacemaker is often required.

Q: Which are the most serious arrhythmias that complicate AMI?

Ventricular tachycardia and ventricular fibrillation are the most common and dangerous arrhythmias that complicate AMI and are responsible for majority of cardiac deaths.

VENTRICULAR TACHYCARDIA

Ventricular tachycardia (VT) can be arbitrarily divided into two categories. If it persists more that 30 seconds or requires termination due to its symptomatology, it is termed sustained VT (STVT); otherwise it is called nonsustained VT (NSVT). Nonsustained type in the postinfarction period is a prognostic marker, whereas the sustained type is not. The QRS complex of VT is typically wide (>0.12 seconds) and occurs at the rate of 100 to 200 beats per minute. VT is further divided into two forms. When the shape of the QRS complex is the same and the rate is regular, it is called monomorphic VT. When the QRS complex continually changes in shape and the rate, it is called polymorphic. Torsades de pointes (twisting of the points) is a form of polymorphic VT presenting as varying amplitude of the QRS, as the complexes are twisting about the baseline. Cardioversion is the treatment of choice in sustained VT. If a patient is hemodynamically stable, drugs such as lidocaine, amiodarone, or procainamide can be prescribed.

VENTRICULAR FIBRILLATION

Ventricular fibrillation (VF) is the most life-threatening arrhythmia and results in disordered rapid stimulation of the ventricles, preventing them from contracting in a coordinated manner, which subsequently leads to asystole and cardiac death if not treated. Ventricular tachycardia usually precedes VF. Routine administration of IV beta-blockers in the acute phase of MI seems to reduce the incidence of serious arrhythmias. Sotalol is of value where recurrent VT or VF has complicated MI. The treatment of choice for VF is DC conversion, with an unsynchronized electric shock with an initial monophasic shock of 200 J, if necessary a second shock of 200 to 300 J, and if necessary a third shock of 360 J. Early use of intravenous amiodarone after failed DC shock can increase the number of survivors.[2] Intravenous antiarrhythmic infusion should be continued for 24 to 48 hours, and urgent referral for coronary revascularization or implantable cardioverter defibillation (ICD) should be considered. Implantable cardioverter defibrillation is similar to a permanent pacemaker, but is capable of delivering a high-voltage shock through leads placed in the heart to convert ventricular fibrillation or tachycardia back to the normal rhythm.

In prophylaxis, the routine use of intravenous lidocaine (lignocaine) in all suspected cases of MI has been discontinued due to its unfavorable risk/benefit ratio. However, intravenous betablocker in the acute phase is known to prevent serious arrhythmias. Amiodarone may have a role to play in prophylaxis.

References

1. Pizzetti F, Tarazza FM, Franzosi MG, et al., on behalf of the GISSI-3 investigators. Incidence and prognostic significance of atrial fibrillation in acute myocardial infarction: the GIIS-3 data. Heart 2001;86:527–532.
2. Blomström-Lundqvist C, Scheinman MM, Aliot EM, et al. ACC/AMA/ESC guidelines for the management of patients with supraventricular arrhythmias. Circulation 2003;108:1871–1909.
3. Kudenchuk PJ, Cobb LA, Copass MK, et al. Amidarone for resuscitation after out-of-hospital cardiac arrest due to ventricular fibrillation. N Engl J Med 1999;341:871.

Index